Charlotte Cooper is a writer whose work has appeared in anthologies, magazines, zines and academic journals. She has worked as a researcher, consultant, organiser and workshop facilitator on fat rights issues. She lives in the East End of London.

Fat and Proud

THE POLITICS OF SIZE

CHARLOTTE COOPER

First published by The Women's Press Ltd, 1998
A member of the Namara Group
34 Great Sutton Street, London EC1V oDX

Copyright © Charlotte Cooper 1998

The right of Charlotte Cooper to be identified as the author of this
work has been asserted by her in accordance with the Copyright,
Designs and Patents Act 1988.

British Library Cataloguing-in-Publication Data
A catalogue record for this book is available from the
British Library.

ISBN 0 7043 4473 4

Typeset in Trump Med. Roman 10/12pt by FSH London
Printed and bound in Great Britain by Cox & Wyman

For my fat genes, inherited via generations of Coopers and Taylors, and in memory of Ro's Mary (1938–87) health professional, mother and dieting partner.

Contents

Acknowledgements

Much love to Simon Murphy/Mona Compleine and Karen W Stimson – your support and intelligence throughout this project has been incredibly sustaining. Thank you Caroline Currey, for helping me through the writing period. A wink to Jenny Corbett, for introducing me to the Social Model. Yvette and David Williams Elliott, thanks for opening new dimensions of activism to me on-line. A special thank you to those who were so generous with information, especially the interview sample. Finally, high fives to my totally cool fat-loving friends and lovers. All right!

Introduction

My Story

I was born in 1968, about the same time as the fat rights movement. I have reached maturity alongside the movement, and this book represents a coming to power for both of us.

Much of my life has been spent trying to come to terms with my fat body. I grew up feeling a deep discomfort that I was, and am, physically different from most people in my life, and this difference was always encoded as shameful. As a young woman I nurtured fantasies of slicing off the fat parts of my body. I dieted, and endured periods of compulsive exercising. I wanted only to see the mythical thin woman who was supposed to be hiding inside me. When it became clear that this ghost was never going to put in an appearance I had to find another way of living.

I first began to think about alternatives to fat hatred as a teenager. My ideas grew out of my nascent interest in feminism and sexual politics, and also, it must be said, from my disappointment with texts that are still considered definitive. I rejected books such as Suzie Orbach's *Fat is a Feminist Issue*[1] because of their false assumptions about fat people. I wanted something more than this.

By the time I began to read books such as *Shadow on a Tightrope* or *Being Fat is not a Sin*[2] I was not only developing a deeper understanding of fat rights issues, but also working through the difficult process of integrating my ideals into my life. What helped and continues to support me was my increasing awareness of a movement of people and organisations who felt and believed similar things, and were actively challenging fat-hating attitudes. As a feminist I was also excited that many of these initiatives were instigated by women. My involvement with the fat rights movement has enabled me to address both the fat hatred around me, and that which existed within myself. It has also given me a space in which to develop my own ideas about what it means to be fat.

Today I feel lucky to be fat. The difference my fatness connotes has been, and continues to be, one of the most challenging and enriching areas of my life. I am very proud of my difference, I feel like a survivor, and I think my perspective as a fat person is a benefaction that has made me special.

Women, Appearance, Beauty and Fat

The fear of fat affects almost everyone. Most people seem to notice some degree of fat hatred and prejudice – it is no secret that fat children get bullied, or that fat women get laughed at in the street. Being fat bestows a status and stigma that most people want to avoid. Weight gain in people of all sizes often signifies disaster; people will do anything to avoid it, and if it were only fat people who went on diets, weight loss industries would have dried up years ago. The fear of fat permeates people's lives as a constant dread that if we do not maintain our bodies we will become a part of that hated group: fat people. The fear of fat encourages people to be judgemental, to put others down in order to safeguard our own precarious status, or to trash our own self-esteem with negative comparisons. The fear of fat is something which controls us.

I am introducing my discussion of fat oppression within the context of feminist arguments about women, appearance and beauty, since they seek to explain our attitudes and anxieties about our bodies, including what it might mean to be fat. Such debates continue the tradition of 'the personal is political' and reframe women's private experiences on to a public agenda. The significance of our appearance is often dismissed as trivial compared to issue X, Y or Z, but how we look, and how we feel about this, has tremendous repercussions. Robin Tolmach Lakoff and Raquel Scherr demonstrate beauty's political relevance in their discussion of the notion of 'Black is Beautiful', which emerged from the American civil rights struggles of the 1960s. They suggest:

> Beauty is never more political than when it is used to prop up the power of one race while it renders others powerless, immured in self-hatred.[3]

For black people living in a culture which encouraged few to really believe this, defining oneself and one's peers as beautiful was an optimistic gesture of defiance and pride, a rejection of prevailing racist values.

Defining appearance as political has entailed allying it to other systems of oppression, such as racism. Hence the term 'looksism' has been coined to refer to appearance-based prejudice. Looksism is a very broad concept which covers many types of bodily difference – that is, bodies which are different in terms of the dominant culture's fantasies concerning normality – and it touches on the intersection of appearance with class, age, race, disability – and fatness.

Looksism supports a culture of beauty which implies that beauty is a desirable goal because it reflects goodness, success, modernity and fashion. Women are identified with beauty and admired for it, our femininity and value lie congruent with it. Feminists such as Wendy Chapkis and Rita Freedman are more sceptical and assert that this culture is detrimental to women.[4] Beauty is a means by which women, downgraded in patriarchal cultures, can bargain for status, and parties who have vested interests in beauty, such as the beauty industry, play up the promises of beauty power. But power awarded on these terms is tenuous; either it reflects only superficial appearances and has little to do with our real abilities, or it is conferred because we have 'played the game'. Beauty is passive, it depends on the beholder to create achievement, and the power believed inherent within it may be false, as even the most beautiful people can still feel disempowered or insecure. Naomi Wolf suggests that women's concern with our appearance is part of the backlash against our struggle for rights, that as we gain power, body anxiety is used by patriarchal culture to keep us in line.[5] I disagree with this position as it treats women as helpless victims without taking into account how we support systems of beauty hierarchies on our own terms, or even how we fight against them. It also ignores the reality that men suffer from body hatred too.

Feminists suggest that beauty is not a natural phenomenon but a social construct, a standard created by patriarchal culture. I would agree that beauty is a construction which depends on many factors, for example class, but that it is not simply a patriarchy which dictates what is beautiful, but any dominant culture to which an individual belongs, as illustrated by the appearance codes of various sub-cultures. However, in being a social construct, beauty is not fixed, standards change, and women are in danger of losing power if we do not keep up, if we fail to maintain our bodies in line with current beauty ideals.

The idea of maintenance assumes that the body is controllable and that beauty is attainable by following certain rules. But because beauty power works by privileging some over many, beauty will always remain elusive to most of us. It is the struggle for beauty which feminists find significant; beauty routines are time-consuming, pointless, they control women as passive consumers, and they have yet more devastating emotional consequences. In *Beauty Secrets* by Wendy Chapkis, a woman called Kathryn discusses her acne:

There are so many little things you have to do; constantly putting on these stupid creams or whatever the latest cure is from your dermatologist. The combination of painful treatment and self-contempt often leads to a pattern of self-punishment. You become completely alienated from your own body. You view it as an unpredictable thing out of control. You disown it. It does not deserve kindness or love. It deserves to be punished.[6]

Freedman believes that such beauty rituals are part of women's socialising process, and feminists are thus critical of the way they encourage women to develop low self-esteem. Traditional ideas of beauty and vanity suggest that women have unfair powers over men, that beauty is an unworked-for, unjustified, supernatural gift. Yet by implying that we can control and develop beauty if we try hard enough, women are caught in a double-bind that makes us damned if we have it, and damned if we don't. Women who do not play beauty games, are not included in, or who reject beauty culture are marginalised and discredited as ugly and undesirable.

Fat Women and Feminist Analyses of Appearance

Feminist discourses around beauty and appearance are relevant to fat women. Fat, like beauty and appearance, can be read in a political context; the stigma attached to being fat is a control mechanism which supports a power structure of one group of people over another, and fat politics is a way of challenging that status quo. Fat oppression is a type of looksism since fat people are constantly judged by our appearance and this impacts dramatically on our self-image and our social status. Many of the arguments outlined above can be set in a context more applicable to fat people by interchanging the word 'beauty' with 'slenderness'. Not everything is so easily translated; for example it is debatable whether slenderness is a social construct. Many of us would argue that slenderness is real and quantifiable, while others would say that the distinctions between fat and thin are blurred and that slenderness only exists in opposition to fatness because it has been positioned as a primary desire in Anglo-American culture – that without such distinctions there would be no such thing as fat or thin.[7]

Fatness, like beauty, is reckoned to be controllable, but as I will discuss later the emergence of set point theory alongside criticisms of weight loss brings this into question. Fat activists, like feminists addressing beauty, encourage people to bring fat issues out into the open instead of veiling them with shame, and seek to change the prevailing cultural values which regard being thin as better than being fat. Within the context of feminist discourses around beauty and appearance, the issue of women being positioned as 'cultural dopes' has big repercussions for fat people. For example, if dieting is being discredited, and if fat is no longer being universally acknowledged as disastrous, how come women still choose or desire weight loss? Similarly, debates about cosmetic surgery have implications as safer fat-reducing surgery becomes more available. Hopefully such arguments can help empower fat people to make informed choices, challenge current medical hierarchies, promote an appreciation of body shape diversity, and celebrate ownership of our bodies.

Although they provide a useful paradigm, feminist discussions of beauty and appearance have failed to engage fat people and fat activists fully concerning the issue of fat oppression. Theories around beauty do not, for example, address health, which is a central aspect of discourses about fatness. In truth, many fat activists feel disenfranchised by these debates. Feminist debates over eating disorders emerged concurrently alongside those over beauty and appearance during the late 1970s and 1980s. Many of these analyses overlap; for example, how the pressure to look a certain way impacts on women's relationship to food, and how this is all a part of the cultural control of women. Both strands also seek to examine women's bodies in a wider social context rather than as a private issue. Many feminist criticisms of beauty make use of eating-disorder theory, but this is awkward territory for fat people as I will discuss later on. Some feminists writing about beauty have failed to question their own assumptions about what it is to be fat, and they promote hackneyed stereotypes. Friedman, for example, comments that fat women express in our bodies an asexual fear of sexuality, and are 'neutered by fat'.[8] Other writers address fatness only to discredit and distance themselves from real fat people. Diamond, for example, adds the caveat:

These arguments do not deny that obesity is seen as a health problem by today's medical standards.[9]

Such statements only further alienate fat women. In other work we are promised representation but in reality are made invisible. For example, in Chapkis' discussion of women and the politics of appearance, a woman called Kathay is cited as being representative of all fat women but tell-tale remarks such as 'when I am fat' or 'when I am thin' make the reader question her status as a fat woman and therefore the authority of what she is saying as a spokesperson. Given women's preoccupation with weight one would assume that in a work which explores women and beauty, fatness would be a central discourse. Yet there is very little specific material about fat women and fat politics other than some photographs and a mention of the *Shadow on a Tightrope* anthology in the Further Reading section.

It seems that feminist analyses of appearance seeking to incorporate discussions of fat women consistently get it wrong! Despite their relevance, perhaps looksism and beauty are too broad a concept by which to examine the details of what it is to be fat. Moreover, fat politics itself stretches out beyond these feminist discussions. Thinner women do not experience looksism and fat hatred in the same way that fat people do, so perhaps it is because these theories are posited *for* us, not *by* us, that if we want to see our lives reflected accurately we should be voicing our concerns ourselves.

My Use of Interviews

Many of the issues discussed within *Fat and Proud* are applicable to all fat people. However, I write with the perspective of a small/medium-sized fat bisexual woman living in a white-majority culture of institutionalised Anglo-American values. This viewpoint is reflected throughout the book, although I try not to assume that my interests are universal. There is not one singular 'fat narrative' but many, often voicing contradictory ideas. To this end I include in my book the opinions and comments of thirteen other fat women, quoted extensively from interviews recorded especially for this project (for biographical details, see the Interview Sample section towards the end of the book). Some of the fat women in the interview sample are known to me as friends and colleagues, others responded to an advertisement I placed in *The Pink Paper*. The sample is mixed in terms of age, attitude, class, ethnicity, nationality and sexuality, although I would have liked to have included more women of colour, and younger fat women, as both groups are severely under-represented in discussions about fatness. All the respondents answered the same questions in person or by postal questionnaire, with some additional follow-up enquiries.

Definitions

There is some jargon in this book, such as 'fat oppression', 'fatphobia', 'super-sized' or 'size-positive', the meanings of which I hope will become more apparent as one reads on. As you have probably noticed, I use the word 'fat' to describe, well, fat people. As far as I can I have avoided using words such as 'large', 'big', 'chubby', or 'cuddly' because they often seem euphemistic to me. Neither do I use 'overweight' or 'obese' because they have connotations of which I am very critical. I realise some people are uncomfortable with 'fat', but for me, using it is about reclaiming a word which has been used to hurt, and substituting its destructive power for a more positive and descriptive meaning.

Who is fat?

There are problems with the various definitions. The standards that define us as fat when we reach a certain weight could be stretched to include, for example, a very muscular 20-stone boxer. The definition that calls us fat when we wear a size 16 or 18 excludes a young or small fat person who fits into a size 14, and in any case dress sizes are not standardised. It might be possible to classify people as fat through Body Mass Index (BMI), a mathematical equation where one's weight in kilograms is divided by one's height in metres squared, or through Waist:Hip Circumference – another standard which seeks to determine whether one's fatness follows an android ('male, apple') or gynoid ('female, pear') pattern. But for some people these classifications support oppressive medical values, and what would it mean for people with a BMI of 29 if a BMI of 30 is considered the universal indicator of fatness? Most often, we define people as fat based on how they look compared to social norms, although this is difficult because social norms vary according to many factors such as region, culture, class or generation. This definition may well be fine for people who are very much fatter than those norms, but where is the cut-off point between fat and thin? What happens to smaller fat people? Who has the right to decide who is and who is not fat? Perhaps it is best that we define ourselves as fat if we believe that to be true. However, this too is problematic since people have different experiences with regard to their fatness depending upon where they are in the size spectrum, and fat may mean a variety of things to fatter and thinner people. In addition, in Anglo-American society most women believe that they are 'too fat', regardless of their size. Amongst this group there are individuals who believe they are fat, yet whose body size is average. I have known women like these glean and contribute strength and energy from size rights initiatives. They define themselves as fat based on shared experiences with other fat people, so are they fat? However, I do not wish to imply that fatness is something psychological; I believe it to be a very real and tangible physical difference. Perhaps it is most useful to define who is fat in terms of experience instead of appearance; maybe we should ask ourselves questions such as 'Do I buy my clothes in specialist shops?' or 'What is my experience of fat oppression?' As I mentioned earlier, there are many fat narratives, so perhaps it is just impossible to make one sweeping definition of who or what fat is.

Obesity

The medical language used to define fatness is troublesome. 'Obesity' is a medical condition named from the Latin for 'having eaten'. It is an inaccurate and misleading definition of fatness since it implies that a fat body is living proof of 'having eaten', that fat in food is synonymous with fat on the body. The predominant belief, in medicine and in popular culture, is that fat people eat too much. This contradicts much evidence to the contrary, including that produced by scientific medical research communities on all sides of the pro- and anti-weight loss divide, as well as assertions made by fat people ourselves. Having our bodies medically classified as having a 'disease' connected with eating misrepresents us, and reduces our lives to an obsession with what we put in our mouths. Furthermore, fatness merely *represents* evidence of 'having eaten'; our perceived greed is a myth projected on to us, it is not real. Yet this symbolic representation is believed to be a hard fact, and is seen to justify our categorisation as abnormal, diseased and discreditable.

Set Point Theory

Despite Orland W Wooley and Susan C Wooley's statement that 'there is *no known cause* of obesity', the categorisation of fatness as a disease carries with it an intense interest in its origin.[10] The popular belief that fatness is caused when a person eats too much, or exercises too little is being discredited only to be replaced by new theories; thus fatness is the result of hormone imbalances, illness, a change in lifestyle. Heredity is being mooted as an important factor – some people are genetically programmed to be fat. Fat people often come from families where there are other fat relatives, and even in cases where diet and lifestyle vary dramatically there can be a genetic propensity to fatness over many generations. It seems incongruous discussing genetics in the context of fatness being seen as a disease, and whilst one's genes themselves are not a type of illness, I would suggest that the notion of there being a 'fat gene' in fat people can be interpreted along the lines of it being an inherited disease, like a time bomb waiting to explode.

Genetics are also implicated in 'set point theory'. Genetic heritage determines our metabolic rate, our ability to transform food into energy, and our 'set point', the body's internal weight-regulating mechanism. Dieting interferes with this mechanism and raises the body's set point which increases one's propensity to fatness. One's body reacts to a diet as though it were starving and compensates by surviving on less fuel. The theory behind dieting suggests that when food is restricted, the body uses up fat cells first and weight loss occurs. However, according to Kelly, this is not so.[11] She argues that since diets occur over a period of time the body does not realise at first that it is under siege and it begins to digest immediate but vital resources such as heart muscle and brain tissue. Only as the starvation continues does the body tap into its fat reserves and body systems slow down. This is the period familiar to dieters as the plateau phase, where weight is difficult to lose and one feels drained and listless. Changes in diet, the end of a diet, or continued yo-yo dieting can result in weight gain as the body protects itself against further periods of starvation. Many fat people have a prolonged history of dieting and attempts at weight loss, therefore it is likely that our metabolisms have been slowed down, and our set points raised. Thus maintaining a steady weight, even one that is high by cultural standards, may be more beneficial for one's health than constant fluctuations.

Set point theory is an increasingly popular alternative explanation of why we are fat, especially amongst fat activists who are critical of weight-loss cultures. It acknowledges a genetic precedent; it accepts lifestyle influences and social pressures specific to fat people, such as dieting; it moves beyond notions of blame and responsibility, where fat people are victims of dieting rather than villainous gluttons; and it attacks diet industries for creating a population of fat people whilst exploiting and denigrating their own market.

Fat and Proud

I have named this book *Fat and Proud* because I want to show that there is honour in the bodies of fat people. In terms of fat politics, fat has many meanings. Being fat signifies being different, being stigmatised and discredited, being hated, feared because we are fat, and being falsely represented as fat people. But fat rights activists believe that fat is something that is normal, part of a continuum of body sizes, and that our positioning in many societies as deviant says a lot about cultural beliefs. Therefore, as a group that is marginalised as 'other', fat people have relevancy and value.

I have opened this book by outlining some key concepts and debates concerning fat people, as well as feminist discourses around women and appearance. I will now go on to identify how fatphobia impacts on fat women's lives, and to discuss our responses to it – from fat hatred through to more empowering responses. A section on health examines some of the ways which are used to define fatness and fat people, as well as some of the 'cures' these categorisations promote. At the end of this section I discuss the impact of medicalisation on fat people, and suggest new alternatives, upon which the final section expands by charting some of the history of the fat rights movement, and its current state of play in the 1990s.

I hope *Fat and Proud* will enable readers to develop some of the ideas already set in motion by fat rights advocates, that this might contribute to a greater appreciation of body size diversity, and that such a move will help all of us to live in and enjoy our bodies instead of fearing them.

Section One

Fat Lives

Chapter One
Identifying Fatphobia

Where to start? I think every day is a hassle, I suppose that's the way I think about it, every morning when I wake up I know I'm going to have difficulties during the day.

Yvette Williams Elliott

Everyday life impacts on fat people in a particular way, often negatively and painfully. Fat people are a social group with shared experiences of the prejudice and oppression that arise in the various situations with which we are confronted. Naming these common experiences enables us to understand the political implications of events we often face alone. It helps us reassess our responsibility for them. Moreover, recognising the patterns, and drawing parallels with other types of oppression, gives us ammunition to fight fat hatred and challenge the institutions which currently profit by our devaluation.

Therefore, in this chapter I have identified some of the situations which show how being fat affects many social interactions, and permeates identities and behaviour. I go on to discuss the wider patterns which indicate that fatphobia is a kind of social oppression similar to racism or sexism. That is why challenging fat hatred entails bringing into question some fundamental beliefs and social institutions.

For thinner people, the knowledge that one physically 'fits in' is usually taken for granted. Contrast this with Karen W Stimson's experiences:

Most of my daily struggles revolve around physical access issues – will the chair/doorway/bathroom/ seatbelt/restaurant booth/etc fit? What alternative and/or advance arrangements do I need to make sure my super-sized body will be accommodated wherever I go today? It's a pain having to check *everything* out in advance and not having access to lots of places and activities – from amusement parks and movie theatres to the corner mini-mart – that ordinary-size people don't think twice about going or doing.

Fat people of all sizes do not automatically assume that we will fit in. We deal with exclusion so often in our lives that we develop ways around it.

At home, to some extent, we can allow for our size and create an environment that is comfortable. Outside, at work, shopping or socialising, many of us have to negotiate inaccessible surroundings. Physical access issues vary from size to size – a place where one fat person fits is inaccessible to another – but the experience of not fitting is common to all. Janne speaks for many fat women when she complains:

> I use the Central Line and the seats on the Central Line are particularly awful. Regular people can just about fit into them; my boyfriend is reasonably slim but he has a hard time getting into them. It's hopeless. I've never been able to sit down on those seats.

Alongside transport, chairs that are too narrow and insubstantial, or seating that is immovable, seatbelts which do not stretch far enough, shops or pubs where the fixtures and tables are cramped together, toilet cubicles, doorways, turnstiles, rides at the funfair, aisles, theatres, cinemas and restaurants are a few of the places where we cannot guarantee that our bodies will be accommodated.

Some places are inaccessible for other reasons. The sheer effort of preparing visits and events in advance, where most people act spontaneously, is enough to hinder us from venturing out. The people who gather or work in some places may have fatphobic attitudes, like the 'Operations Manager' at London's Stringfellows nightclub, who comments:

> The majority of fat people have great difficulty in dressing appropriately. They don't take as much care with their appearance as slim people. Invariably that means that fat and sloppy people are refused access to the club.[1]

Exclusion can be an embarrassing and humiliating experience, so we avoid areas where it is likely to happen.

Fat people have difficulties finding clothing to fit. Whether we want to dress stylishly, or whether we need uniforms, or special protective garments, size is the main issue. The clothing industry is deeply conservative when it comes to stocking and sizing garments. Where larger sizes are available they are often more expensive, especially when they are included within the same style range as smaller sizes. Most clothes shops operate a policy which covers British sizes 10 to 14; some include size 8, others have expanded to sizes 16, 18 or 20. Specialist large-size retailers, or concessions in some chain stores, have a wider range, but not all the sizes are represented throughout all the styles. Few retailers stock clothes above a size 30, although some smaller shops will make up a design to order, for a price. This means that super-sized people, particularly those on low incomes, have considerable problems in finding clothing to wear. Karen W Stimson comments:

> I make most of my own clothes (even undies!) if I want to dress 'appropriately', 'fashionably' or even comfortably.

The recent introduction in Britain of a few more large-size clothes shops has generally passed by super-sized people. Also, smaller fat women are now focusing attention on issues which have become more important than the availability of sizes, such as choice, quality, cost, ethics and design. Caroline Currey remarks:

> There's so much talk about consumer satisfaction nowadays, and yet we're completely invisible and treated like sitting ducks . . . I don't want to walk around in diaphanous t-shirts and trousers. The mail order catalogues use slim models. As consumers we're not seen.

Shopping for larger sizes remains an event segregated from the mainstream, and fat people feel stigmatised. We do not have anywhere near the choice of clothing that thinner people enjoy, and many of us continue to subscribe to an ethos of 'if it covers me up, I'll take it!'

Fat people are culturally invisible. Recently there has been an explosion of interest in the role of the media, its effect on fat people, and the way a culture responds to fatness. This interest focuses on two areas. First, the mass media presents a limited vision of normality where fat people are under-represented. Many argue that because of this we suffer from a lack of validation and helpful role models. Certainly our invisibility reflects the way our lives and needs are often disregarded. Secondly, representations of fat people in the media tend to be insulting. Here are a few recent examples. One writer was 'disgusted' by the fat people spoiling his summer holiday by 'polluting' his beach with 'hillocks of flab'.[2] He believed the sight of fat people was 'certainly as offensive as any crap floating in the water'. Television critic Victor Lewis-Smith commented about a woman 'so fat she could have fallen down and not noticed it'.[3] Another columnist remarked of a fat woman too frightened to leave her house: 'If she did she would be the only man-made object on Earth, besides the Great Wall of China, to be visible from outer space.'[4] And in political cartoons fatness is often a metaphor for greed, corruption and stupidity – the cartoonist Riddell of the *Independent on Sunday* and the *Observer* produces countless examples of this.

Much of the speculation around media issues has been concerned with how negative references to fat people create stereotypes and reinforce fat-hating values. There is some disagreement about this, partly because there is rarely a consensus about who or what constitutes a 'positive' or 'negative' image, and partly because there is no acknowledgement of images or performers that fall into both camps. In discussions about media representations and stereotyping many of us refer to a kind of 'brainwashing' effect. The idea is that culture is so saturated with negative imagery that as readers, listeners and viewers we have become overloaded and are unable to use our minds, or to make our own decisions. Some academics argue that the 'bombardment' theory is too simplistic in that we are not easily manipulated but are actually sophisticated and critical media consumers. I do not wish to get caught up here in a debate about whether or not the media is able to brainwash us, only to say that being invisible or witnessing gross distortions of our lives without the power of redress is part of the low-level buzz of fat hatred.

In our private lives families and friends often regard our bodies as open targets. Even within our closest relationships we receive messages that there is something wrong with us, and we attach feelings of blame, guilt and failure to our fat bodies. Comments and assumptions can be intolerable, undermining our confidence, and leaving us mistrustful of those we love. Many of us grow up with family 'teasing' and fat-related nicknames, which can position us into painful roles. Some of us have been fat all our lives, we come from families where fatness is our genetic heritage, whilst others are 'the odd one out'. In all types of family, young fat people are often exposed to the fat hatred of their parents, siblings and extended relations. Ellen asserts:

> My family are very fatphobic. My mother in particular is obsessed with her (extremely low) weight and takes a very punitive approach to fat people. She once advised me to buy my clothes a size too small so that the constant discomfort would remind me to diet!

Not all families are overtly hostile, but many operate a hidden agenda where even 'kind' remarks can be devastating, as in Yvette Williams Elliott's experience:

> . . . some of the things that my parents have said to me, meaning well, meaning to help. You know, I can't claim that I have terrible parents, I have wonderful parents, I love them, but without realising it they have said things that have come back to haunt me. Very often, I think everyone has this feeling sometimes, a memory comes back so vividly that it feels as though it has just happened. There are certain incidents that come back to

haunt me. If I'm feeling slightly vulnerable that day they can be enough to ruin the whole day or keep me indoors.

In other families the issue of a person's fatness may be considered as a shameful embarrassment which becomes a taboo subject. In many cultures, traditional family values enforce rigid patterns of parental authority, which can make it impossible for young people to question fatphobic attitudes. Most fat people start weight-loss programmes as children, and patterns of dieting and body hatred can survive through many years before they are challenged. Sometimes, long into adulthood, we never question these early messages.

Being fat has repercussions throughout our public lives. Many of us have painful experiences of harassment by teachers and other pupils at school. Later, being fat makes us vulnerable to negative attitudes which prevent us from finding work or gaining entrance to higher education. Some employers assume that a fat body connotes that we are not fit and healthy enough to do the job, that our presumed poor health will lead to high levels of absenteeism, that we lack self-control or an interest in our appearance, that we are not worth employing because there will be no uniforms to fit us, or that we will not reflect the corporate image, especially if it is 'sleek', or has recently been 'slimmed down'. I myself have lost work for some of these reasons.

For fat people work can be limited by weight restrictions, such as those enforced by some airlines, or we might find ourselves hidden in backroom jobs, where there is little chance of us working with company clients or the general public. As in the outside world, the working environment can be physically inaccessible; toilet cubicles too small, chairs too narrow. Some of us have to deal with prejudiced comments or non-verbal disapproval from our colleagues and managers. This is not always intended as overtly hostile, but that does not mean that the underlying values and assumptions are not offensive to us. At work it can be difficult for us to challenge comments, especially if we are outnumbered, outranked, or if the people making them are unaware that they are being insulting.

The behaviour of work colleagues reflects the way people respond to us in the wider sense. Fat people receive a huge amount of unwanted attention. We learn to read stares and whispers indicating everything from disapproval to horror and disbelief. As fat women we are public property, as though our bodies were made to be commented upon, especially where our eating habits are concerned. Viv Wachenje recalls an event with her late husband:

> I remember once we were on holiday and we'd gone into a cream tea shop. There was a very large woman having a cream tea. He got worried about that, he said 'I don't want you ending up like her.'

Many of us will not eat in public because of the 'plate watchers' who police our appetites; that is people who comment or make non-verbal judgements about the type of food we eat, and who layer their observations with fat-hating assumptions. For example, Germaine Greer watched:

> . . . a hugely obese German mother push aside her delicious Italian meal, snatch up the chocolate ice lollies that her children had abandoned on the table and literally push them one by one into her face. Under the table her vast thighs were moving spasmodically in a grotesque version of orgasm.[5]

Long after such comments are made, eating in public can still be fraught, as can shopping for food, and social occasions at which food is central.

Our bodies are presumed to be funny. In December 1992 the British broadcaster and television producer Jonathan Ross wrote and presented *Fat*, a programme about food and popular culture in America, which featured much footage of fat people unknowingly being filmed. During *Fat* Ross described us as 'big, fat, dopey, simple friends'. In a promotional interview he argued:

> I don't think we're being cruel, even to obese people. They're fat and they're stupid, but in a nice way.[6]

Perhaps it is this kind of prejudiced paternalism which underpins the sneers Max Airborne has to endure, such as:

> constant harassment from men and kids. This is especially compounded by the fact that I drive a motorcycle, so people seem to think they have an extra reason or right to harass you. It gets worse when I'm driving with my fat girlfriend on the back.

Mandy mentions that she often finds 'people pointing me out to their friends'. Lee Kennedy has similar experiences:

> I get more people screaming out of cars lately, that seems to be the thing. Sort of loud maniacal laughter out of cars passing by. And stares too, of course, always stares.

More frightening is when laughter gives way to increasingly threatening behaviour. Janne experiences:

> hassle from kids and men mainly. From kids it's 'fatty' and staring and gawping at me. It can escalate to throwing things at me.

Sometimes the abuse she suffers is sexualised:

> Because I'm big I'm going to have big breasts and, you know, 'look at those big ones' or 'fat arse', or things like that.

On occasions the abuse intersects with other aspects of our identities. For example, Janne explains that as a woman of colour some of the fatphobic harassment she encounters is also racist.

Being different in some way from an assumed norm makes fat people super-visible and vulnerable as targets. We find that people consistently invade our space without our consent with comments or non-verbal messages. It is as though we are always expected to be accountable for ourselves whatever the stereotype that is projected on to us. We are seen as objects of disgust ('Ugh, how did you get so huge?'); suspicion, or scorn ('why are you eating that, aren't you fat enough?'); we are patronised as pathetic victims; or as one-dimensional super-positive role models. We are expected to react, to apologise, to have comebacks, to be 'strong', to assimilate the invasion. Paradoxically, although our bodies make us highly visible in the physical sense, on other occasions we are completely invisible, for example, when we are overlooked as potential partners and lovers as though our fatness counts us out. Being invisible means that our needs are left unmet, for example, access issues, or even just understanding, or they are overlooked as ridiculous. When our feelings and reactions count for so little in terms of everyday fat oppression, it can seem as though we do not exist.

Many people now know that it is unacceptable to be overtly hostile to fat people, it is seen as 'bad manners'. But this does not prevent some from mouthing sentiments such as 'she's fat but she has such a pretty face', or 'I feel fat and ugly', where the underlying values are still fat-hating. The message always gets through. Amongst our interactions silence, collusion and exclusion are almost always assumed. It can take enormous courage for fat people to speak out; we risk ridicule, disbelief and denial from those who refuse to treat us as anything more than a tolerable joke, and who believe that our distress has nothing to do with them.

Fatphobia can operate in more subtle and demeaning ways. Some comments are intended as compliments – for example, that our fatness makes us more feminine than thinner women, or more 'emotionally stable', that it indicates that we are more likely to put our family and relationships first, or that we are more fun to be with. I feel uncomfortable with these assumptions because they are based on the view that all fat women are alike, and that the way we behave is determined by the fat on our bodies, rather than our personalities, or our experiences of fat oppression.

Fat people are found in every social strata but we are not one homogenous group. Being fat impacts differently on particular social groups, and our identities will determine the kind of fatphobia we suffer. Some groups have developed tools for fighting fatphobia, for example, out of their experiences of ageism. Many older people are critical of cultural values which place a great emphasis on youthful beauty, and the emerging disability rights cultures have been very effective at condemning exclusive standards of attractiveness. Fatphobia also combines with other body image issues. Those who contravene social norms concerning 'appropriate' appearance, such as women who have had mastectomies, or disabled people, will also have a different experience of being fat. Perhaps such people will have developed their own strategies for dealing with fat hatred as a result of coming to terms with other aspects of their body image. But difference does not protect anyone from internalising the same fat-hating beliefs as everybody else, by which I mean taking dominant cultural values on board and acting upon them as your own beliefs, especially since, unlike a mastectomy for example, fatness is considered reversible, a personal choice. Moreover, fat people are not validated by the same support networks as people with other bodily differences.

Fat Women of Colour in Anglo-American Culture

Black cultures in Anglo-American society sometimes do not suffer as virulent and institutionalised a form of fat hatred as many white cultures. Joan Dickenson mentions positive portrayals of fat black protagonists by black women writers saying, 'Only rarely do white characters even be *fat*, let alone talk about it.'[7] Some types of body fat are acceptable on women in some communities, for instance in East London where I live big bottoms and thighs are desirable amongst young working-class Afro-Caribbean people, whereas slenderness is the universal rule for white women. Age also has an impact; it was found that a sample of fat black women aged between 66 and 105 were two and a half times more likely to be satisfied with their weight and to consider themselves attractive compared to a similar group of fat white women.[8] Many black women reject Barbie-like standards of white beauty, which also entails rejecting slenderness as the epitome of attractiveness. Donna Allegra comments:

> I certainly embrace big-bodied women and have no desire to look anything other than an African woman. I reject the 'skinny blonde' ideal as the only image of beauty.[9]

However, not all people of colour have a positive race identity, and this might impact on one's self-image as a fat black woman. Fat hatred still exists. In communities with a less hostile attitude to fatness, fat-hating medical values are now taking over and weight loss is becoming more prevalent. Such communities are not exempt from the influence of media, fashion and advertising, which inform medical attitudes, and weight loss for minority cultures is also posed as a means of assimilation into the dominant culture. Some personal accounts by fat black women do not fit with the assertion that black people are more accepting of fatness. In *Shadow on a Tightrope*, for example, a woman called Deb talks about the cross-generational fat hatred in her family, the criticism she deals with as a fat person from her mother and younger sisters. According to Sondra Solovay, in 1993 William Tingle, a black deputy district attorney of Alameda County, California, prevented three black women from taking up jury service. Whilst it is unlawful to discriminate against jury members on the basis of race, other factors are acceptable, and Tingle objected to these women because they were too fat and dressed in a way he did not like and considered 'radical'. In a newspaper interview he remarked: 'Young, obese black women are really dangerous to me . . . I've never liked them and I think they sense that.'[10] The appeals court supported his decision.

Perhaps there is an unwillingness amongst black communities in predominantly white cultures to acknowledge fat hatred. Some black theorists and activists make the same judgements about fat people as does the dominant white culture – for example, Adams, an academic writing about black women's health, reiterates the standard disease model about fat being unhealthy. Such communities are already under attack from racism, they do not want to make themselves more vulnerable, or diffuse their energy on 'lesser' issues, including fat hatred. Asserting that the marginalised community has the answers to the dominant culture's problems is a mark of pride, it demonstrates that there are positive aspects to different communities. So it could be regarded as painful and embarrassing to acknowledge that black and white cultures do share similar problems around their attitudes to fat people. Indeed, regardless of attitudes towards fatness and fat people within one's ethnic community, fat people of colour still have to interact with white cultures and white fat hatred.

Stereotypes

Fat hatred combines with racism and as a result fat black women suffer different stereotypes from their white counterparts. For a long time the Mammy figure was, for the white population, the acceptable face of black womanhood from the American Southern tradition, from slavery and the Civil War. As a loyal and passive servant to white people, she was usually depicted in the kitchen around food. The Mammy was bossy and cantankerous, stupid and non-threatening. She was the comic relief: jolly,

self-mocking, outrageous and unsexy. Her body was played
for laughs when she stamped, wiggled and danced. The
Mammy will be familiar from films such as *Showboat*, *I'm
No Angel* and *Gone with the Wind*.[11] Here the central
white female characters are presented as the epitome of
beauty, and the fat black woman as the embodiment of
black ugliness. Different actresses interpreted the Mammy
in different ways. In a lecture about Hattie McDaniel at
London's National Film Theatre in 1994, Stephen Bourne
said: 'She breathed life into a stereotype and infused roles
with integrity and depth. She interpreted them as
assertive, flamboyant, and tough.' Yet the stereotype
endures and still affects fat black women's identities
today. Donna Allegra remarks:

> I don't want to fulfil that role. My stance here parallels
> why I never ate watermelon as a kid: it was expected
> that I would just love watermelon and grow up to be
> Aunt Jemima, fat and cooking happily for whites. I
> bridled fiercely against satisfying a stereotype no one
> will admit to holding.[12]

Racist myths influence other stereotypes of fat black
women, particularly the 'sexy mamma' which plays off
fantasies about black women's sexuality; the skinny black
woman as hard, mean, infertile, unloving; and the fat
black woman as loving, nurturing, full of life and passion.
Other stereotypes start out as role models. The sassy,
belligerent and loud 'strong black woman', exemplified by
singers such as Bessie Smith or The Weather Girls, seems
positive because she is not passive, but exuberant and
larger than life. Dickenson mentions that some of us
'counteract the degraded image of fat black women by
idealising it', calling on a 'tradition of strength, of power in
both mind and body',[13] and Mason-John interviews Sandra,
a woman who 'enjoys the strength and power of being a
very big black woman. Nobody will threaten her, and she
feels completely safe walking down the street late at

night.'[14] However, the notion of strong black womanhood has impacted on other fat women in different ways. Anna Johnson remarks:

> Even as a black woman I am sometimes viewed by others as someone who is just slightly angry and difficult. I was even referred to by a former black colleague as an *'intimidating* sister'. There is absolutely nothing in my nature that would lead to that opinion: I am warm and friendly and speak in a calm, low voice. I can only assume that this erroneous impression is brought on by the fact that I am a 'large' black woman. As someone who wants more than anything to be liked, this attitude is rather unsettling.[15]

To which Honorine Woodward responds:

> Part of it, I think, is the societal stereotype of the Black Matriarch, but part of it is likely that we are articulate. Let's face it – we mutually have *four* Others here: color, gender, size and orientation – and when the Other finds a voice, people get scared.[16]

Perhaps stereotyping is the cultural response to vocal fat black women whom it would prefer to stay silent. Such representations are not as vitriolic as many images of fat white women, but this does not automatically mean that they are 'positive', since they all force women to behave in a contrived way in order to gain acceptance.

Racism
Fat black people need support in areas which do not seem so pressing for fat white people. For example, issues around mental health are pertinent, since black people are disproportionately represented throughout the mental health system. On the one hand normal behaviour, such as anger, is labelled by professionals as abnormal when it involves black people, which is very similar to the way

that all fat people are pathologised. But on the other, racism and fatphobia play off each other, causing and feeding on self-hatred and depression, which can lead to coping strategies such as eating disorders and agoraphobia. Racism also impacts on white people, Allegra asserts:

> White women are kept in line by racist devices as well – their beauty measured by how much they don't look like people of color. We are said to wear the characteristics, like weight on a woman's body, that are deemed unacceptable by white American beauty standards.[17]

Acknowledging these issues not only enables the fat rights movement to extend its support, but also to develop its understanding of fatphobia. For example, older black women occupy the fattest, and also one of the poorest, socio-economic stratum in Britain, and this has important implications for activists challenging fat hatred in terms of class and medicalisation. Including ethnicity, alongside a host of other identities, into the movement is beneficial to us all.

Naming Fat Oppression

Being fat affects ordinary areas of our lives, but because of their everyday nature we sometimes think of fatphobic attacks as trivial and random. Once we begin to acknowledge that there are patterns and similarities throughout these experiences, and that they happen to all of us, we can begin to make sense of what we once regarded as isolated incidents. When patterns repeat themselves over and over, we find it helpful to name that phenomenon in order to distinguish it, and understand what purpose it serves.

I regard fat hatred as being congruent with other forms of oppression. Like racism or homophobia, fat hatred is part of a complex web of social power relations and hierarchies where particular social groups are marginalised, stigmatised and discredited. Oppressed groups find that information about them is distorted, or denied, that assumptions are made, and stereotypes promoted. People who are oppressed suffer from prejudice.

Like other kinds of oppression, fat hatred plays on divisions between people. It encourages us to think in terms of binary oppositions, by which I mean that the fantastic variety of human body shapes is reduced to two opposites: fat and thin. This is a mentality which, given two choices, will assume that one must be superior to the other; hence thin is better than fat. It is a dry and colourless distillation of the marvellous diversity of human body shape. Furthermore, fat hatred is a power system in which we are all losers by various degrees, as it exacts an enormous cost on people of all sizes. Where fat people are reviled everyone will continue to live in fear of becoming fat, experiencing body hatred and insecurity. But the cost to fat people by way of self-hatred, shame and victimisation is insufferable. I would suggest that much of the behaviour that is regarded as appropriate for fat people, for example, being self-deprecating or embarrassed about our bodies, is not inevitable or 'natural'; it is a response to the social expectations and pressures that are put upon us. These manoeuvres are all focused on a personal reaction, and reinforce the mistaken belief that fat oppression is an individual's issue, and that the responsibility for change lies with fat people.

Challenging fatphobia is problematic. Despite its casualties, the preservation of the fat-hating status quo is paramount. Fatphobia in twentieth-century Anglo-American societies is replicated and underscored by some fundamental cultural institutions and power bases such as the media, where representations of dieting and preoccupation with weight are seen as 'natural' for fat people. The free market economy likes to sell us a never-ending stream of profitable weight-loss dreams, and in a later chapter I discuss how medical science has a vested interest in furthering fat hatred. All of these institutions influence our values and beliefs. Because these institutions and beliefs are powerful, most people do not have the resources to rebel against them; and because they capitalise on common and familiar anxieties, many people do not question their aims. But ending fat hatred entails challenging these cultural foundations, and being able to accommodate alternative viewpoints and politics. Many people gain by our powerlessness, and lose when we become powerful. It is in their interests to perpetuate the myth that fat hatred is normal, trivial, or the fault of fat people ourselves, all of which makes it very difficult for us to rock the boat.

Chapter Two
Responding to Fatphobia

Few fat people glide through everyday difficulties without a reaction. In this chapter I will describe some of our emotional and behavioural responses to living within fat-hostile environments: fat hatred, fat acceptance and fat activism. I begin with some of our more common reactions, such as anger and self-hatred, and then move on to find different ways of negotiating fat oppression which work upon elevating rather than demeaning our self-esteem.

Fat Hatred

Blame

As fat hatred is an everyday occurrence it is difficult to distinguish between the constant stream of negative messages, and the truth based on real life experiences, which often contradict the mythology. For example, I have always been a very active person. As a child I enjoyed swimming and riding my bicycle, and today I love to walk, go dancing, play-wrestle, and feel strength and movement within my body. However, I have only recently remembered this, so caught up have I been with assumptions that all fat people are lazy and passive. It is confusing and distressing when our self-knowledge does not tally with what our cultures are telling us about fat people.

By accepting cultural attitudes about how greedy we are, or how offensive our bodies appear, fat people learn to feel responsible for the oppression we suffer. Thus, when clothes don't fit, we feel responsible; when someone comments about the food we eat, we feel humiliated; when the seating is inaccessible, we are embarrassed because we know that it is our fault we are not thin enough to fit in; when members of our families make demands on us to lose weight, we feel guilty for not being what they want us to be.

Many of the interview sample remarked that fat oppression made them feel angry; from what Kristine Kay describes as 'a momentary pissed-offness', towards the anger that Lee Kennedy experiences as 'sort of thwarted anger, you know, simmering', through to downright rage. Even when we direct our anger outwards, we often put ourselves under increasing pressure to speak out at every injustice. However, sometimes it is not possible to respond, perhaps it will make things worse, or put us in danger. The infringement of our space, somebody screaming abuse out of a car window for example, is often set up in such a way that it is impossible to respond. Sometimes we blame ourselves for not confronting people. Max Airborne explains:

> Often I get angry – sometimes I confront things on the spot, sometimes I don't and I berate myself afterwards for my cowardliness.

For Karen W Stimson:

> Depending on how strong I am at the time and/or how much support I have, they can make me mad enough to do something or crumple into a ball of depression.

Like Ellen, we find ourselves making decisions about the possible effectiveness of answering back:

> It makes me feel frustrated and tired. I'm always evaluating whether it's worth the bother of confronting someone's prejudice.

In having to decide whether or not to confront people, Mandy, like many of us, often feels self-conscious, under attack, aggressive and guarded:

> *Mandy:* I like to make people aware of what mother-fuckers they are, and even just to make them out to their friends to look like idiots. I know it's petty.
> *Charlotte:* Is it 'get them before they get you'?
> *Mandy:* Yeah, pretty fucked-up really. I want to get out of that.
> *Charlotte:* But I guess you have to be ready for things, otherwise you can be hurt.
> *Mandy:* I'm always on the defensive. I think a lot of people just kind of wear blinkers to do what they've got to do, but I'm always looking out for stuff.

Dealing with blame, confusion and anger on a daily basis can leave us exhausted. Even when there is no overt abuse the fear of conflict can affect our lives intensely. Many of us want to retreat, like Max: 'Often I am just plain tired of it and want to hibernate in my room.'

We withdraw to places where we feel physically and emotionally safe; some of us experience panic attacks when we are out in the world and we become agoraphobic. In my own experience it has sometimes felt much easier to stay at home for days, no matter how isolated I become, than to go out and deal with a potentially hostile environment. Many women in the sample mentioned their experiences of depression. Frequently these feelings were attached to factors such as dealing with sexual abuse, living in poverty, being tied to low-paid and boring jobs, and experiencing body hatred, rather than specifically about living with fat-hating abuse, although everybody complained about having to negotiate such mistreatment. I have heard some sufferers refer to mental distress as 'anger turned inwards'. When the source of abuse is thought to be the fat person's own body rather than oppressive social attitudes, the frustration and despair experienced combined with anger can lead us to abuse ourselves. Some women develop coping strategies such as eating disorders and practising or fantasising about self-harm; indeed some writers and fat activists might suggest that dieting and weight-loss regimes are themselves a form of self-harm. Fat hatred teaches us that we are ugly, gluttonous monsters who deserve nothing better than the discrimination and abuse that we suffer. As fat people are considered culpable for such abuse, we believe that by taking responsibility to change ourselves, to lose weight, to become smaller, fat hatred will no longer happen to us. Max Airborne comments:

A lot of my dieting wasn't by choice, but when it was, I'd say it was due to the constant pressure from my family and the world at large, compounded by the fact that I'd internalised society's hatred of fat. Feeling unhappy and blaming it on being fat because that's what I was always told.

Many fat people also experience an ambivalent and uncomfortable relationship to food because of the intense scrutiny our appetites are under. An example of how fat people's eating habits are the focus for obsession concerns my nephew Sam. Coming from a family whose genetic inheritance consists of many fat people, and some big broad men, Sam himself is large for his age, and his appetite is cause for anxiety. At a recent birthday gathering one of the older relatives commented disparagingly, 'No wonder he's so big, shovelling that food away.' Sam is one year old, he has only just learnt to walk, and already the obsession is starting. Many fat people share a history of dieting which in itself distorts the values we place upon eating. Some of the problems we experience because of the cultural fixation on our appetites, and because of the culture of weight loss, are feelings that we are not entitled to food, that we should deny ourselves pleasure and nourishment. Sometimes we feel embarrassed by our unruly appetites, and we compensate by eating in secret, or not eating at all.

Losing Weight

Fat people are fat because we eat too much, it is our fault; if we don't like fatphobic abuse we must lose weight, it is our choice to make, we have no grounds for complaint. In twentieth-century Anglo-American industrial cultures we are encouraged at every juncture, via all media, throughout many institutions, by experts, by people we trust, to believe this. So we do.

Weight-loss programmes, such as dieting, surgery, even therapy, all of which are discussed more fully later in this book, bring with them particular sets of emotions. Sometimes we feel coerced by the false promises of how losing weight will transform our lives, as in Mandy's experience:

They made me feel depressed, fucking pressurised, like 'once you lose that weight you're going to be one fabulous person'.

These promises are offensive, implying that we are somehow deficient as we are now, but Caroline Currey identifies a strong trend which runs throughout dieting emotions, which plays on our desire to escape our fat bodies and embrace what Yvette Williams Elliott later names a 'golden future'. Caroline remarks of her diets:

They all had novelty value and most of them made me feel extremely euphoric because I lost weight with most of them and that always induces a high. The flipside was that I'd come down and they'd make me feel terrible. The weight *always, every single time*, would go back on again.

For Yvette the euphoria of losing weight was mixed with uncertainty and anguish:

Always a rollercoaster of emotions. It was that terrible up-and-down between hope, powerfulness and strength when you felt that you really could do it, hope for this golden future that you thought you were going to get, followed by complete despair, self-loathing, being convinced that I was a morally, and in every other way, deficient person. Generally speaking, the hope and joy was only a very tiny percentage of it, self-loathing made up the rest.

Inevitably there would be the comedown. Max Airborne experienced depression and says that the weight-loss programmes she followed left her feeling:

Sick. Physically, emotionally and psychically awful. Diets put me in a downward spiral of self-hatred. Worthless. Incapable of achieving success.

For Annette Cooper, semi-finalist of Weight Watcher of the Year, dieting left her feeling:

> Out of control/useless/greedy/disgusting/pathetic when I binged. I felt moody/irritable/obsessed with food as a general rule, and hopeless when the weight went back on.

Janne followed some very low-calorie diets which made her ill:

> I was fainting all over the place. It made me feel awful, because obviously you can't keep it up for more than a week or so, so it made me feel a failure.

Even when we 'succeed' there is disillusionment. Karen W Stimson recalls:

> Nothing much changed, except that my mom was able to buy me some pretty clothes from Spiegel's mail-order catalogue. My school grades went up in gym but down in all my academic subjects (I was an A student before) and I started obsessing about food for the first time in my life. The kids who made fun of me before I lost weight still didn't like me and didn't consider me 'thin' even though I was considerably smaller than I'd been. My friends were still my friends.

Camouflage

Fat people might not be actively trying to lose weight, but wanting to appear smaller and more socially acceptable can still be a goal. There is a terrible pressure to be 'normal' or invisible which undermines fat people's feelings of security about our bodies. Shouts, stares, comments, and the 'usual stuff' mark us out as monstrosities and leave us, like Lee:

> Just feeling like a mega circus freak. Desperately trying to hide myself all the time.

Our physical presence becomes something that is embarrassing or shameful to us. Sometimes we harbour desires of becoming invisible, 'normal', of escaping, or wanting the ground to swallow us up. Janne remarks:

> It makes me feel that I wish I wasn't this size. When you just go in the street and get nothing but being stared at and nasty comments the whole time you're out, I wish you could just blend into the crowd and just be anonymous.

Some of us celebrate our rejection of normality in other areas of our lives, but difference is a liability when it is framed in terms of being fat. Lee Kennedy attests:

> Oh yes, [my lifestyle is] my choice, that's the way I want to be, I suppose. I just don't want to be abnormal as a freak, as a physical freak.

Sometimes we try different methods of fitting in, alongside, or instead of, dieting. Clothing is most often used to help us 'pass' as thinner, to disguise ourselves. We might put on elaborate corsetry, and wear only certain clothes of a particular 'flattering' style, or 'slimming' cut, or 'waist-skimming' length, clothes that disguise and hide our bodies. Passing in this way translates into a series of clothing rules with which many fat women are familiar. Women's magazines in particular often publish lists of 'Dos and Don'ts' which come in and out of fashion, such as avoiding horizontal stripes, or encouraging the use of large shoulder pads 'to balance the figure'. Away from specialised lighting or soft-focus camerawork, and in spite of our apparel, it is impossible for fat women to look very much smaller. However, for the wearer, clothes and practices imbued with the belief that they help us fit in and radically alter how we look are a significant psychological survival manoeuvre.

Other times we try to pass by dissociating ourselves

from the very notion of fatness itself, for example, many fat people will not tolerate any discussions of fatness, and some deliberately distance themselves from other fat people lest they be viewed and judged together. Perhaps we feel that if we refuse to identify as fat then we will not suffer fat oppression.

Some fat people try to create compensatory personalities 'in spite of being fat', in the hope that it will be our qualities that are noticed instead of our bodies. Fat people can become trapped in roles, such as being the life and soul of the party, self-deprecating, a super-achiever; or practices, like always wearing elaborate hairstyles or immaculate make-up and clothing to distract attention away from our fat bodies. These make us unable to be our natural selves. For others, the mythology of fatness is so painful that many of us seek to remove ourselves from it altogether by denying ourselves basic physical require-ments if we think they will contribute to a stereotyped vision of us – for example, refusing to eat in public even if we are very hungry, or trying not to breathe heavily or gasp for air when undertaking strenuous physical activities. Both of these are attempts to contravene the image of fat people as greedy, lazy slobs. But fat people have as much right to be greedy, lazy, unfit or smelly as thinner people. By wanting to present only what we feel is positive and acceptable, we deny our human limitations as though they were a terrible affliction, as well as the chance to accept the help that we need.

The possibility of passing, trying to lose weight, wanting to become 'normal', is about the only recognised option available to fat women in twentieth-century Anglo-American culture. Large-size clothes shops, for example, sell long, draping garments instead of the fitted and body-conscious fashions that are prevalent along the rest of the high street. When we follow clothing rules instead of wearing what we want, it is as though we are communica-ting our desire to look 'normal' or 'presentable', but trying to camouflage our fatness implies that the reality of our bodies is too terrible to admit. It is a futile gesture. Passing does not threaten the status quo but denotes passivity and resignation, this is why it is socially sanctioned. Passing may be an attempt to make a place for ourselves in a fatphobic society, but it is a denial of who we are and what we look like. It is a placatory gesture to a society which hates fat people, it shows the culture which wants us to disappear that we are 'trying to do something about this awful weight', whatever the cost to our well-being. Passing will never be empowering; as individuals it will never make us look small enough to be granted acceptance and power as a thinner person, and as a social group there is no chance of achieving meaningful social change when we are caught up in self-denial.

But there is an alternative: fat acceptance and fat activism. Fat acceptance is an individualistic response, whereas fat activism is a more collective rebuttal. Both overlap and are mutually supportive.

Fat Acceptance

Fat acceptance is characterised by a deep and lasting acceptance of our bodies whatever our size. When we feel proud and strong we find ourselves hurt less often, and giving ourselves permission to be fat with no recrimina-tions generally makes us much happier. Feeling good helps us change old patterns: we stop wanting to lose weight, we lose our faith in dieting, and we prefer to treat our bodies with warmth instead of viewing ourselves as objects to be punished.

Fat acceptance is a slow and ongoing process and is different for everyone; some women are unable to approve or celebrate their fatness, others may find that they have been working to find peace with themselves before they even knew what they were looking for. We tend to find our own way. We live in cultures that are saturated with negative messages about fatness, which are internalised to some degree. It is easy to challenge things that are unusual, but to question beliefs that are familiar is perplexing. Challenging the status quo entails risking many things, and an enormous social pressure tries to keep fat people silent and compliant. It is miraculous that anyone ever begins to question the fatphobic mythology that surrounds us, but we do.

Sometimes we experience a sudden change in one part of our life which enables us to reconsider our attitudes to fatness. Yvette Williams Elliott recalls:

> Going to college gave me a language that helped me to think about things. I find I think that theorising things is very much a double-edged sword; sometimes it's helpful, sometimes it isn't. For me it's always been helpful, it's been a way of reaching an accommodation.

Even in our closest relationships our fat bodies are often too taboo to discuss, so when emotional patterns in our personal lives improve, perhaps when we enter more supportive relationships with people, this can be revelatory. Coming to terms with fat hatred in the past is another part of the process which enables us to move on. Many of us have experienced negative family attitudes regarding our bodies, schoolyard insults, and other fat-related hurts and humiliations. Working through past grief can involve unravelling a tangle of coping tactics. Referring to the early trauma she experienced as a fat child, Jean Midson comments:

> I've recognised those as childhood things and patterns that you develop, kind of safety strategies that you can use to protect yourself.

Other areas of our lives, for example work, can also be influential. Sometimes we witness events which challenge us into altering our own assumptions, like Viv:

> Working here I have been aware of mothers who want to

control their daughters through weight control, and that really interests me. Seeing that kind of attitude started to wake me up.

Some of us begin to integrate fat rights into our lives by combining it with other beliefs and frameworks we might already have, as with Karen W Stimson's experience:

My activism sparked when I made the connection between sexism and sizeism (though that word hadn't been coined yet) back in the late 60s/early 70s. NAAFA [National Association for the Advancement of Fat Acceptance] referred to 'civil rights' for fat people, and my hippie/leftist/feminist consciousness went into overdrive.

Often it is a series of things which wake us up, and not one particular point. Karen recalls:

Being rejected for admission by the first three colleges I applied to despite excellent grades, references, Honor Society etc. And when I finally got into a university, they wouldn't let me into their secondary teaching program because the dean thought I was 'too fat to be a teacher'. So I graduated with honors but without that vital teaching certificate, and couldn't get a job. Bingo: one size rights activist is born!

Many of us find that we can no longer accept the painful events and memories which accumulate, so we decide to try a new tack.

In the past such change would inevitably involve losing weight. However, as dieting is increasingly discredited, we have begun looking for alternatives. For Caroline Currey size-positive theory made more sense to her than years of dieting, she now has:

A deep belief that's matured over the years that this is for real. I think when I was dieting my belief in dieting was always quite tenuous, it was like holding a magic talisman. But my belief in set point weight theory and everybody having a comfortable weight is deep, deep, deep, deep down.

The growth of the fat rights movement has also created a context within which people who hold similar beliefs to Caroline can now find support.

Coming Out Fat

When ideas spark inside our heads it is like the first stage of coming out. This is an expression traditionally associated with sexuality, but it often refers to those who make public an identity which is largely invisible and discredited in the wider society, so coming out is also valid for fat people. Coming out as fat means that we no longer want to accept the general belief that there is something wrong with us. By coming out we begin to acknowledge our bodies as normal, acceptable, even worth celebrating, instead of hiding and denying ourselves. Coming out makes us visible, it shows that we are fine as we are. It is a personal step which has wider social and political consequences, such as the promotion of diversity.

There are many ways of coming out, including privately to oneself, by acknowledging one's body in photographs or in the mirror, by challenging comments and being open and talking about fat; and more publicly, by not being silenced when the seat is too narrow or the clothing won't fit, or by being open and talking about being fat amongst friends and colleagues. Coming out involves identifying and accepting certain issues as having relevance to our lives, instead of pushing them aside with horror or embarrassment. For example, Lucy began to put herself in the picture because:

It started with the growing realisation that diets don't work, and opening a copy of Shelley Bovey's book *Being Fat is not a Sin*, seeing one of Lee Kennedy's wonderful drawings and thinking 'oh my gosh, that's my life!'.

Coming out enables us to get and give support. Many of us find that we welcome the companionship of other people going through the same thing. Annette Cooper tells of how a book provided the ignition for her interest in fat rights issues, but that her activism blossomed when she began to connect with other people.

Fat is a Feminist Issue started it. I know it has its critics but it was the very first time I heard anyone challenge the system. It had never occurred to me it could be done. It was such a revelation. I then started my journey of self-worth looking for anything else to build on my new found way of looking at things. Then the Fat Women's Conference started the snowball effect. So much *power* in the group. And I suppose the last big influence was running assertiveness and women's development workshops for the last three to four years.

Coming out is an ongoing process that begins with challenging our beliefs about our own bodies and continues as we search for support and recognition throughout our relationships, and in society. It is a major step towards making peace with ourselves, which for some of us may develop into activism, and recognising ourselves as part of a community.

Whilst coming out as a fat person and being fat-positive are often mutually compatible, is it possible to be fat-positive and not have come out? Yes, if that person supports the notion of fat rights but is not fat themselves. This might also be true for a fat person who does not identify as fat, or perhaps they are 'in denial'. Conversely, some individuals are out as fat people but their behaviour could be described as fat-hating; Rosemary Green consistently derides fat people, including herself, as being 'horribly diseased'.[1] Generally I find it difficult to label behaviour 'fat-positive' or 'fat-negative' since these terms have different connotations for everybody.

Fat acceptance not only impacts on our personal

identities but also on the wider context of our lives. Instead of taking on the values of dominant cultures and feeling threatened by or abusive of fat people, we begin to understand why as a minority group we are scapegoated and marginalised. We gain a sense of commonality with each other and a recognition of our shared experiences. Many of us begin relationships with fat people as friends, lovers, colleagues or political allies, perhaps coming together to share our strength and knowledge, to develop ideas or for mutual support. Perhaps we decide, when we can, to use and buy products and services that are relevant to us, and support businesses or organisations which recognise and celebrate our existence.

Fat Activism

Most of the interview sample view themselves as fat rights activists, some are members of fat rights groups, and some are founders of such organisations. Others had not considered themselves activists before answering the questionnaire, since they assumed that 'activist' indicated a person who, for example, attends demonstrations or leads groups.

Fat activism is an individually defined expression. I take it to mean the directed behaviour of someone who has reached a certain accommodation of their own fatness, or of other fat people, someone who has a certain consciousness of what being fat might mean, someone who wants to change the status quo, and someone who speaks out to effect social change. Becoming a fat rights activist entails taking some responsibility to create change. Caroline Currey's decision to be out and active as a fat woman stemmed from:

. . . the fact that there are not many fat activists. If on every street corner people were dropping out of diet clubs, and on every street corner there were women saying 'Diets are rubbish, any sort of even pseudo-diet is

rubbish, anything to try and lose weight is rubbish', I'm
sure I'd just sit at home and I wouldn't bother to do any
of these things. But because there are not many people,
I do.

Most often activism is conscious, although some of us do
things and hold opinions without knowing there is a
context and a precedent for them. Janne says:

I didn't really understand what [fat activist] meant. I
went to the Fat Women's Group last week and it was
really great to hear what they'd been doing. It was the
first time I went and I really enjoyed myself. But I don't
think I'm a fat activist right now, I didn't even know
there was such a thing, I'm afraid. I knew there was stuff
in America, I know they've got the NAAFA and I've seen
it on Oprah Winfrey a couple of times, but in this
country I didn't know there was anything at all, really.

Fat people often struggle with feelings of low self-
esteem, and the experience of ridicule, harassment and
abuse can inhibit us from making a noise. Yvette Williams
Elliott comments:

I think I have a very difficult approach to political
activism. I'm not good at demonstrations because I'm
too frightened. I think that they are vitally important
but I'm scared stiff to go on them, so I rarely manage to
get myself to appear in the right place at the right time
behind a banner, even though I'd like to.

Therefore, as fat activists we take these risks and fears on
board and tailor our activism to meet our own needs and
resources. Few of the interview sample take to the streets,
but many act individually. Caroline Currey's activism is
typical:

I write and complain about ads, or if I see something on

television, or hear something on the radio, any sort of media that I feel is promoting anorexia or ridiculing fat people, I write and complain. I also speak up socially when fat issues come up, and that can be a lot more difficult. But quite a lot of the time when I speak up, my anger fuels me and I don't just let it ride. I let a lot of things ride, but not fat issues.

In this way we can do as little or as much as we want, tailoring our activism to the environments in which we live and work – Yvette, for example, includes fat rights issues on the syllabus she teaches. For activism to be effective, it needs to reflect our abilities, and take into account difficult situation. Annette Cooper:

I always deal with comments on a one-to-one basis. The only time I don't is when I am in a crowd with no one person to direct it to, eg I'm in a public place, hear a comment (negative) from a group, but don't know who said it. I haven't had the bottle for that yet.

Fat activism is not for everybody but the ability to challenge fat hatred is crucial to our development of fat-positive self-esteem – Annette remarks that 'not being quiet!' helps her feel strong. It demonstrates to outsiders as well as to ourselves that fat hatred is unacceptable, and enables us to develop assertive strategies to deal with fat hatred, which in turn help us to feel validated. Annette concludes that speaking out 'gives me power. I am not a victim'.

Part of my support for activism is that it effects a collective change whilst simultaneously achieving the more personal benefit of self-empowerment. Activism can be approached in a variety of ways, there is no one method. This gives us a choice about how we want to respond to fatphobia, whether it is by ourselves, or through organisations we join or create. Activism can be as imaginative as we want it, or as accessible and everyday.

Being activists also connects us to a long tradition of protest for civil rights around the world. It is an optimistic endeavour, and it is comforting to be reminded that others have set a successful precedent for change.

The notion of activism begs the question: can you come out and not be politically active? Many people have a block on what they perceive as 'political' action, they regard it as something other people do, as humourless, dictatorial, worthy, judgemental and dogmatic. Sometimes it is. Sometimes over-zealous activists promote a condescending view of fat people who do not identify as they do, as though they assume a moral authority, and as though they represent all fat people. For fat people who do not identify as activists, such attitudes generate feelings of guilt for letting the side down, or resentment for being pushed into something against one's will. Political activism in the traditional sense of petitions, direct action or group organising is just one way of effecting change, it has roots in a particular kind of culture and may not be relevant or accessible to everyone. Upon coming out or developing self-acceptance as fat people, political activism may not necessarily be the ultimate goal, and not every out fat person with a positive self-image would define themselves as a fat activist – as I have said activism is an individually defined phrase. However, the notion of activism also depends on what is defined as 'political'; just walking down the street could be contextualised as a political act when we are encouraged by fat hatred to stay hidden away. Self-acceptance, our private lives as fat people, is often read as being outside culture, outside politics, but I do not believe this is so. I think that whilst body size has such social resonance, whatever we do as fat people will have some political repercussion, no matter how small the act.

Chapter Three
Living Fat

So how do we *really* feel about being fat? Most of us acknowledge that there are two ends of the spectrum; either we feel very positively towards our bodies, like Kristine Kay:

> I'm always happy! I don't know if I'm stupid, my head's under a bag, or something, but I never get that unhappy about myself. It's like 'Well, this is who I am, so what's the point of being unhappy about it?'

Or, like Lee, we do not:

> How do I feel about myself now? Not good. Really horrified.

However, for many of us our self-image of our fat bodies is not as simple. Certainly, fat rights issues have made a huge impact on our lives, but we continue to experience complex and contradictory emotions. Many fat women have decided to reject dieting and self-hatred, to embrace a more accepting attitude towards our bodies, but whereas diets and weight-loss fantasies offer a quick fix to our problems, fat acceptance is a much longer haul, and living fat presents contradictions.

Still Wanting to Lose Weight

Although some fat people have decided to stop dieting, and may be vociferous in our rejection of dieting, many still wish to lose weight. Cancelling our membership to Weight Watchers does not prevent us from self-monitoring our calorie and fat intake, or secretly buying diet food, or even just wishing.

Given their interest in fat rights issues, it may come as a surprise to learn that most fat women in the interview sample still desired weight loss to some degree. Many of us assume that it is incompatible to be a fat activist whilst continuing to harbour hopes of losing weight. However, we live in the real world. Weight loss is still a considerable aspiration; how could it not be when we receive so many cultural messages about the value of thinness over the horror of fat? Lee Kennedy remarks that she wants to lose weight unreservedly:

> Desperately, really desperately. I just feel like my whole face is lost, just swimming in blubber, and I want my tits removed totally.

However, Lee's answer was atypical from the rest of the

sample, whose desire for weight loss occurred by degrees tempered by their knowledge and acceptance of fat rights issues. As Jean Midson says: 'I do want to lose weight but I am not going to diet.'

For some, weight loss is tacked on to other goals, such as overcoming eating disorders. Sometimes we harbour fantasies of becoming ill and 'just happening' to lose weight, or else we neglect ourselves with the hope that we will become thinner. Losing weight in this manner also enables us privately to assimilate negative values about fatness without appearing to be fatphobic. Sometimes we construct our desire to lose weight as a side-effect because it is painful for us to acknowledge that we are still unable to accommodate our fat bodies, or admit that we want to be thinner, since there is much shame around fat activists wanting to lose weight. Yvette Williams Elliott explains:

From a feminist activist point of view I think there was a lot of emphasis in the 70s and the 80s about accepting yourself, and I think that's what I initially hoped – that when I stopped dieting I hoped I would be able to accept myself and I haven't been able to. I think it's very difficult to do that when things are constantly thrown in your face by your everyday experiences. But I do feel that somehow I should have been able to do that, and I feel guilty that I haven't. I feel that in some very obscure way I am selling out by still wanting to lose weight, because I have strong political views about ideologies of beauty being oppressive to women.

That many of us still want to lose weight, in spite of our commitment to fat rights, is a painful issue. Not only do we make ourselves vulnerable to the very diet industry of whom we are critical, and the whole host of weight-loss proponents that we are trying to question and distance ourselves from, but there is also pressure within the fat rights movement. Fat activists who want to lose weight are regarded as people who have sold out, or undermined the arguments for self-love and self-acceptance which underpin the movement. People who acknowledge fat rights issues yet still want to lose weight are caught in a new web of shame and guilt.

Some of us want to lose weight because we are concerned about our health, for example, Annette Cooper says:

> I would like to lose some, purely on the basis that I want to live long, and not be crippled by arthritis. If it weren't for that I would not.

Fear of fat-related ill-health is very strong. At the root of this fear are the cultural messages we receive about fatness and its connection to ill-health, which are amongst the most pernicious myths about us. These myths are often the most difficult to question. Until we have access to healthcare that is free of fatphobic mythology fat people will continue to have fearful relationships with our bodies, and will always negotiate health in terms of weight loss.

The weight-loss ideals of fat women in the sample are not about being transformed into supermodels. Yvette Williams Elliott explains:

> My fantasies of being smaller have changed considerably over the years. I think now about being small enough to fit into a cinema seat. I do not think about being a size 12 any more. I wonder how much weight I would have to lose before I could sit in that seat and watch the film and be comfortable. That is the epitome of my ambition rather than 'I want to look like Naomi Campbell', which I'm never going to do, and probably wouldn't want to anyway. I think my ideas about what is acceptable have actually expanded, even if they haven't expanded enough to include me the way I am now.

Instead, these desires are pragmatic in the context of living in cultures where, for example, there are considerable physical barriers to surmount. Some of the interview sample explained that it is living in a society where we are undervalued and hated that makes it most difficult for us to feel positively about our fatness. Karen W Stimson lists some of the social barriers:

> The constant ubiquitous physical barriers I have to deal with as a 400lb+ woman with impaired walking mobility. The attitudinal barriers that enforce fatphobia and size abuse. The economic and social downward mobility which have resulted from my oppression as a fat woman. Not having access to health insurance or unbiased medical care. The attitudinal barriers are almost as bad. I'm tired of having to educate EVERYBODY! I just want to be treated like a human being.

No matter how good we feel about our bodies, we still live in environments where there is pressure to lose weight. Mandy expresses this dilemma:

> I feel good most of the time but there is the constant reminder that I don't belong. I hate conformity but it seems the only way if I want peace and happiness in my life.

Therefore we balance between conflicting ideologies which some of us, like Karen W Stimson, try to evaluate:

> My mobility and some size-related health problems (eg arthritis), would be improved if I weighed 350 instead of 400lb+. But that's not going to happen naturally, and I'm not going to further exacerbate my health problems by going on a weight-loss diet. I recognise that the stress of oppression (and physical barriers to access, plus lack of access to healthcare), is the biggest contributor to my health problems.

As fat activists we try and redirect our anger and dismay towards fat-hating cultural attitudes, but sometimes we still end up back at square one, blaming our bodies for our oppression and feeling overwhelmed by our fatness. Lee Kennedy:

> Knowing that people find me disgusting, and being the butt of loutish humour and what-have-you hinders me from feeling strong. I feel trapped, hopeless, just so over-burdened with weight that I'll never be able to shift it.

Some fat women in the sample answered that they did not want to lose weight, although their answers were conditional. Referring to her dreadful experiences of dieting as 'that knife-edge and that nightmare scenario', Viv Wachenje does not want to lose weight 'because I'm happy with myself now'. However, she adds:

> I'm not saying there are bits of my body I wouldn't like to change, but they're as much to do with having had two children, having a less-than-taut stomach, things like that. I think well, you know, that's my landscape.

Ellen does not want to lose weight:

> Although I do not want to gain any more. If I *did* lose weight, I suppose I'd be pleased at some level, but it's not a goal that I'm trying to achieve. I guess I have to admit that I still have internalised social pressure to lose weight.

By outlining such conditions to ourselves we are acknow-ledging how difficult it is to release completely the desire to lose weight, and challenge the values which surround that desire.

Given the evidence that fatness is genetically determined, and given the fallibility of weight-loss techniques, becoming thinner permanently is not a realistic option. However, weight loss remains an aspiration that is defined in dream-like, wishful ways. Like a fairytale, slenderness will improve our lives by some indefinable way, it will be the happy

ending to our everyday problems. But Mandy has looked
beyond the rainbow to consider how she would really feel:

> I go crazy thinking about the way people would change
> toward me if I was to lose weight. I don't think I'd be able
> to handle it. It's like: 'Fuck you, you wouldn't have
> accepted me when I was fat, so why should I give you the
> privilege of my presence now?' I'd also be screaming from
> the inside saying: 'Look at me now, this is how you want
> me to look and you don't even recognise the difference'.
> Just being slim and thinking: 'Come on, you know, I'm
> slim now, reward me, or do something because this is
> how you want me to be, why aren't you acknowledging
> it?' Obviously they're not going to, they don't know you,
> so what are they going to say?

What if we try to imagine what would really happen if we
lost weight. What would it be like living in a different body
after we had struggled so hard to find self-acceptance as a
fat person? How would we feel about people commenting
or not commenting about our thinner bodies? Would we
have to maintain such a body? What would this entail?
Would it damage our health? Perhaps we would feel as
though we could no longer depend on the support of the fat
rights movement. Maybe we would feel insulted that
people who once ignored us were now showing interest. We
might feel that an essential part of ourselves had been lost,
as though a limb had been amputated. Losing weight would
not wipe out all the things that had happened to us as fat
people. Caroline Currey comments:

> If a fairy said: 'By magic I can turn you into a naturally
> slim woman', I'd be very tempted. I think my value as
> a fat woman that has been through a lot of bad
> experiences with trying to change her body shape, and
> has come largely to terms with her body, actually
> makes me quite special and quite valuable, and I hope
> I'd tell the fairy to take a jump.

Perhaps it is helpful for us to consider our fantasies of losing weight as a temporary stage which it is possible to surpass. Maybe we can find strength in trying to separate the dream from reality, and acknowledging that we come from places where our bodies are hated. Perhaps we can learn to appreciate ourselves not as victims of society but as survivors.

Fat activists who want to lose weight are living a paradox by embracing oppositional ideas, and still believing against all the evidence to the contrary that we can and should exert a choice regarding the size of our bodies. Whilst some people work through such contradictions towards a more solid self-acceptance, others live permanently with these inconsistencies. After all, life itself contains many contradictions, it does not come processed in perfectly wrapped ideological packages. No matter how much we revile our fat bodies, or struggle to integrate fat acceptance into our lives, what is important is that we can still glean strength and support from fat rights initiatives. Lee:

> I'd like to regard myself as a fat activist but obviously I consider myself very much a victim of my size. There are other rules for other people. I've always had this thing, like other people can be healthy and good-looking though fat, but I'm different. I think there's a limit to how fat you can be before it gets bizarre, and I'm past the limit as far as I'm concerned – although I really approve of fat rights zines at the same time. It's contradictory.'

Rethinking Blame

Size acceptance does not make us immune to the things which make us depressed or unhappy, but one of the most significant things we learn from fat rights issues is the ability to contextualise our problems and negative feelings. We stop blaming ourselves for feeling ugly or unworthy, and instead try to consider the social attitudes which encourage us to feel bad and ashamed in the first place. Max Airborne asserts:

> I feel a lot better about myself than ever before, but sometimes I look at myself and I'm shocked and horrified, so obviously I still have a lot of self-hatred to overcome. It's so deeply ingrained! It's still hard for me to fully enjoy receiving sexual affection, even though I want to. I still wear certain clothes because they hide the truth of my body. My ideal thoughts and my feelings aren't always in sync. with each other. Mainly I hate the world for having such hateful, stupid, petty attitudes about beauty and bodies. I often feel like an alien, despite the fact that I have a significant community of other fat dykes around me.

Karen W Stimson is also pragmatic. She adds:

> I have bad days and good days, but they're related more to my accomplishments than to what my body looks like (though my failures seem connected, often, to the fact that I have always had to battle size abuse and discrimination when trying to accomplish *anything*!). I have a fat aesthetic when looking at other fat women and men, and I like the way my body looks, the way it moves, especially naked. I don't like it when I'm squeezed into too-small seats or the door to the bathroom is so narrow that I can't get in, but that's society, not me. Still, I get depressed regularly.

Fat acceptance helps us create more imaginative responses to fat hatred. Some of us have learnt to sneer back. Max Airborne says:

> Sometimes I laugh at people for their stupidity and feel secure in the knowledge that I am a better person for having gotten past such bullshit. But interacting with the world requires a lot of strength and frequent pep talks.

The strength and resilience with which we face the world can be empowering in itself. Viv Wachenje's reactions have changed for the better:

> I think some years ago comments from friends would have upset me a lot more than they do now because I've done quite a lot of work on myself, just learning to value me as I am. They don't wound me quite as much, but of course they still can. I don't think you ever get completely immune to people's comments, I don't think it's possible, but I'm more able to think 'well, why did they need to say that?' instead of thinking 'what's wrong with me?' That's the stage I'm at now, it's really their problem and not mine, it's beginning to shift a bit in its focus.

Jean Midson has become more resistant. When people complain that she is obstructing their way she is philosophical:

> I suppose as I've got older and more enlightened I think 'well, tough'.

Elsewhere we have built safe communities for ourselves. Max Airborne explains:

> The fact that I have many fat dyke friends helps – at the very least I can create social situations where I'm around people who 'get it' and I can feel free to be my fat self.

When we get together with our fat friends we often have the confidence that we lack when alone, which can help us feel rebellious, playful and proud when our difference is pointed out; we are worth staring at!

> Mandy: I don't like eating on public transport or walking down the street because I think people will look at me and think 'oh God, no wonder she's so big'.

Charlotte: But also I've been with you when you've eaten publicly as an act of defiance. Do you remember in Crouch End when you ate that big sausage roll? People were going past you going [shocked expression], and you were going [big smile]! It was really cool.
Mandy: That's true.

Reconciling past problems and acknowledging the difficulties of living fat enables us to build new horizons for ourselves, like Janne, who feels:

Most of the time pretty good. I'm dealing with the abuse because it has a direct relationship with my size. It can really bring me down sometimes but its getting a lot better. Coming out as bisexual has been really good. I've got somebody who really cares about me, my boyfriend, and other friends I've made since I moved here. I just feel a lot better about myself. When I used to be at home they'd be putting me down all the time about everything and I just had zero self-esteem. At least now I can complain about things and feel like I'm a worthwhile person most of the time. It's a hell of a lot better.

Realising that things are actually getting better helps us appreciate how far we have come. Caroline Currey says:

Nowadays my self-image is consistent. That's miraculous after twenty years of going up, down, fat-me, thin-me, fat-me, thin-me. I am now slowly beginning to get a stable self-image. I guess I feel like a battle-scarred survivor, and very proud. I think I've worked through a hell of a lot.

Feeling Good

Often we have to make a conscious effort in order to feel all right. Viv Wachenje explains: 'Sometimes I do have to do a bit of mental gymnastics to get myself back into being

"Well, I'm okay".' Feeling good also entails learning to recognise those things which help us feel strong, which takes practice. Despite ambivalence about our bodies, and despair at having to live in cultures which are hostile to fat people, many of us enjoy areas of our lives where we feel validated. The support of our lovers and partners, for example, who see us in our most private moments, who care about us when we are feeling raw, vulnerable, strong or beautiful, can make a great impact on our self-image. Yvette Williams Elliott explains:

> I think being loved has made me feel tremendously strong. I think that in the past I have been very reliant on my partner but he has enabled me over the years to move forward on my own. I wonder if it hadn't been a lover, if it had just been a friend, would it be the same; just that experience of meeting someone who really liked me unreservedly, not 'I'd like you more if you were thinner', but 'I like you, you're fine!'

For many of us, the relationships we have with other fat people are deeply significant. Feminists have discussed women's friendships with each other as places that are powerfully affirming and offer a private space in which to work things out. Not all of our friendships are intensely fulfilling, and they often generate the same problems as any other relationship, but being with other fat women, trying to support each other, acknowledging our bodies, or playing with our similarities, is profoundly liberating. Some of us enjoy 'touchstone' relationships in a more public setting, for example, in groups.

Being in touch with the way our bodies look and feel helps us feel good. Lucy enjoys cultivating her image:

> I love having new clothes as well as old favourites. I recently accepted a job mainly because I didn't have to wear smart clothes (and fail miserably with the power dressers and Laura Ashley set). To be honest, I always

struggled against the idea that fat women should wear understated coverall dark colours (no frills, no stripes etc). I love bright colours and flamboyant stuff, but never really had the nerve to wear it until a friend of mine said, 'I think you're a bit of a drag queen'. After I got over the shock of being 'outed' I thought 'what the hell, yeah!' I've been much braver about what I've worn since then (although I'm still working up to the pink satin number!).

For others, being physically fit is a means of generating an appreciation for our bodies. Max, for example, finds that 'swimming and other forms of exercise' help her feel strong, and Jean Midson finds pride in 'the fact that I feel well. I don't get silly trifling illnesses. I recover quickly when I am ill.' Sex, too, is a wonderful way of connecting with our bodies! Acting on desire and pleasure can give us a new respect for the way we look and feel.

As fat women we take up space, we are not easily budged, so knowing that we have a strong physical presence is a source of pride. Kristine Kay suggests of her physicality that:

There is some sort of comfort in that I can move about and go places that most women might be afraid to go. I don't really think about it, maybe it's stupid, and maybe some day I'm going to have the mother of all muggings happen to me, but people don't tend to mess with me. I think it's because I cut a more intimidating figure.

Many fat women are caught in between self-loathing and self-acceptance. Some will develop a more solid acknowledgement of our bodies, some might 'regress', feeling that progress is too slow, that we have made an effort, and that nothing can really change the way we feel about ourselves. Most stay 'inbetweenies', presenting an outward image of self-acceptance but retaining many traditional social convictions, for example, a faith in the authority of medicine, or particular attitudes towards women, femininity and beauty which tell us that being fat is unhealthy, ugly and makes us unlovable. It is tempting to read these responses as stages, with acceptance as the pot of gold at the rainbow's end. However, our lives are more complicated than these categories suggest, and we might find ourselves flitting from one attitude to another. Therefore I suggest we regard these response patterns as parallel, not linear, since each one has different risks and benefits.

Unlike the empty promises sold by weight-loss proponents, there is no diet or single answer that will transform our lives from sadness and self-hatred to empowerment. The fat women from the interview sample have explained some of the things that worked for them. Often these seem insignificant and tangential compared to the 'real' struggle. The size rights movement provides a base from which to develop. However, the key in our personal incorporation of fat rights issues is that we are realistic about what works for us, and that we find our own pace, and our own rewards, rather than conform to orthodoxy or political dogma.

Section Two

Health

Chapter Four
Danger! Obesity!

During any discussion about fat oppression there are inevitable references made to health. Common sense tells us that fat people are unhealthy, it is an irrefutable fact. The dangers of obesity have been established and recorded in the most controlled and meticulous way by generations of scientists, and the disturbing evidence has since filtered into the collective consciousness. An ever-growing charter of ailments, from trivial to fatal, are caused or exacerbated by an overweight body: heart disease and disorders of the circulation, arthritis, back pain, flat feet, skin complaints, mental illness, diabetes, early death. The research findings, the charts, the statistics and the reports are all proof.

How do fat people confront such unassailable 'proof'? I have already mentioned that challenging fat phobia effectively entails questioning familiar but deep-rooted beliefs about some of twentieth-century Anglo-American culture's fundamental institutions. Our arguments about the relationship of health to fatness are based on what we think we know about issues such as disease and the neutrality of medical science. What we accept as the objective truth is more likely to be the result of a complicated system of cultural attitudes and values.

Disease

'Obesity' is a medical condition named from the Latin for 'having eaten'. Obesity is considered a disease because a fat body is regarded as proof that somebody has eaten too much according to social norms, and eating more than one is thought to need is considered pathological; gluttony is one of the seven deadly sins, after all. For optimum health it is believed that the body should utilise all the energy it consumes. When food energy is transformed into fat in the body it is hoped that this will be a temporary measure, that the fat is merely 'stored' for future use, although a small amount of 'surplus' is acceptable in women since this is necessary for menarche. If the fat is not used, or 'burnt', through physical activity, its long-term presence indicates that the body is not coping efficiently, so the fat body is therefore diseased. Obesity is regarded as a disease that affects the body by inhibiting its essential functions, for example the heart and circulation, and puts one's health at risk by increasing the chances of contracting other ailments. Different degrees of obesity confer varying levels of attendant risks. This is exemplified by the medical terminology for obesity which has several strata with which to catalogue differently sized fat bodies, from 'overweight' to 'morbidly obese'.

When we define fatness as a disease we are acting within powerful social boundaries which control what we believe to be right and appropriate, or shameful and abnormal. In many contemporary cultures disease is taboo, a reminder that we are primitive and mortal. Much of our sense of progress and modernity is based on the pride of our rational and scientific triumph over diseases which previous generations suffered from and attributed to random Divine punishment. Yet even in the modern world we retain fantasies about the meaning of illness – we have brought the disease upon ourselves for example – and ill-health continues to be read as a metaphor, perhaps a symbol of some unnameable moral failing.[1]

Society depends and thrives upon order, predictability, strength and maximising the potential of our bodies by maintaining good health. Disease represents disorder, chaos, weakness and badness; it inhibits our ability for optimising our lives, both as individuals and as members of a culture. There is a social stigma attached to disease that expresses itself through avoidance, fear and mass panic over threats of epidemics, contagion and infection. Disease is repugnant – to think of our fat bodies as diseased is so threatening that the language we use to describe our fatness, such as *surplus* or *excess* weight, or *over*weight, is suggestive of some weird growth that is separate to the rest of us. We call fat unaesthetic and ugly. Indeed, the prospect of always being fat is deeply disturbing, with many of us insisting that our fatness is merely a temporary blip in our otherwise slender lives.

Whereas disease in the distant past was contextualised as a supernatural punishment, modern Anglo-American attitudes to disease reflect many of the founding tenets of twentieth-century capitalist society. Some of these beliefs underpin the work ethic of rewards for honest labour, the belief that a person is responsible for their own destiny and that we exert a free choice over our bodies, whereby illness is considered to be a personal failing, and health a triumph. In terms of religion and Christian-based spirituality, if one's physical body is regarded as a Divine gift fashioned in the image of its Maker, to be thought of as an abuser of that gift is sacrilege. As in the work ethic, we believe honest toil always rewards us, therefore the drudgery of a diet will furnish us with a healthy and slim body. Values inherent in this desire are obligation, will-power, control, discipline, a focus on individual achievement, competition, conspicuous activity – and guilt if we do not perform what is expected of us. In contrast, we fat people are thought to have let ourselves go, to have ignored these rules and therefore must suffer the consequences. Richard Klein asserts that in Anglo-American culture, fatness represents a craving for oral pleasure and satisfaction that is believed to be self-destructive.[2] This is particularly reprehensible of us when the rest of the culture is working so hard to keep in shape, and it leads us to the notion that our immoral conduct has led to our physical ugliness.

Defining fatness as an abnormal and temporary state is damaging. First, it sets up a corresponding belief that thinness is the only true healthy normality, a fascistic value which negates the possibility of there being validity in bodily difference. Secondly, defining fatness in terms of disease promotes the idea that slenderness represents stability, but in reality the opposite is nearer the truth. Slenderness can be an extremely precarious state for many of us, especially when dieting creates dramatic fluctuations in our body weight. Thirdly, since disease is loaded with negative connotations, and health with positive ones, to regard fat people as diseased entails thinking of us as abnormal and bad, and thinner (although not very thin) people as healthy and virtuous. This impacts on fat people's self-image through guilt and embarrassment, and promotes a belief that we must lose weight to become acceptable. Slenderness is also linked with survival; if we don't lose weight we will die. Fat individuals are seen as pitiful or morally corrupt for what is believed to be our imminent yet preventable abandonment of our loved ones.

So what are the health risks of being fat? According to *Obesity*, a report by the Royal College of Physicians, diabetes, gall-bladder disease, hypertension, arthritis, respiratory problems and cancer have increased incidence in fat people.[3] However, this report uses height/weight tables based on insurance company statistics to define 'obesity' and, as Shelley Bovey points out, they have included weights which might be considered 'normal' as 'overweight', and thus their definition of who and what is fat is open to interpretation. Bovey argues that being moderately fat, not more than two stones over the height/weight charts, is healthier than being underweight, and the Royal College of Physicians found that the lowest mortality rates were found in 'mildly obese' middle-aged people. Whilst Susan C Wooley and Orland W Wooley suggest that it is 'highly doubtful' that there are any hazards in 'mild obesity', they believe that there are some health risks associated with being very fat, such as maturity-onset diabetes, osteo-arthritis, and, in super-sized people, respiratory disorders such as sleep apnoea.[4]

Let us try and unravel some of these statements. Fat people may experience an increased risk of developing late-onset diabetes, but Paul Ernsberger and Paul Haskew argue that this is a less serious form of the disease than hereditary diabetes, and they go on to say that fat people have a more favourable prognosis for diabetes type II than thinner people.[5] Fat people are at risk of developing respiratory disease, but Ernsberger and Haskew contradict the Royal College of Physicians and Wooley and Wooley to say that fatness is associated with lowered incidence of some of these types of disease. According to Bovey, fat women are at increased risk of developing endometrial cancer, but Ernsberger and Haskew engage in a complex discussion of the many statistical risk factors surrounding cancer, and suggest that, overall, there is a lower mortality rate for cancer amongst fat as opposed to thinner people. Fat people are at an increased risk of developing osteo-arthritis, but Bovey presents evidence that arthritis is affected by weight, not caused by it. Fatness is most often cited as a risk or causal factor in coronary heart disease, but this link is also ambiguous. Wooley and Wooley add the caveat: 'Even if correlations are found between weight and certain diseases, this is not, of course, evidence of a causal connection. Both may be due to an unknown third factor' – heredity, lifestyle or dieting, for example. Bovey found that fatness by itself is less a factor in coronary heart disease than age, sex, blood pressure, smoking, lifestyle and raised blood fats, and Ernsberger and Haskew assert that there is a lower mortality rate amongst fat people who have high blood pressure or coronary heart disease than amongst thinner sufferers. Naomi Wolf also points out that in the US, the National Institute of Health study linking fat to heart disease and stroke was performed on men. She states that in 1990 similar studies on women found that there was a fraction of the risk. It appears, then, that some fat people are at risk of developing some forms of diabetes and some respiratory diseases, but that medical research presents no blueprint; that there are a great many lifestyle factors to be considered, and that nothing is certain. Let me add that being fat, even very fat, is not an inevitable recipe for disaster, it does not automatically guarantee that we will develop these problems. Ernsberger and Haskew point out that there are even health benefits to be gained from being fat – statistically, fat people experience a lowered incidence of osteoporosis, fractures, anaemia, some types of diabetes, peptic ulcers, scoliosis and suicide. We have an increased immune system and a lower fatality from infectious diseases when compared to thinner people. Fat women are less likely to have to deal with eclampsia in pregnancy, giving birth prematurely, vaginal laceration, hot flashes or premature menopause.

The real risk to fat people's health is in our attempts to lose weight. Furthermore, the stress of living with stigma and prejudice causes its own health problems and, interestingly, many of the diseases attributed to fatness, such as high blood pressure and heart disease, are common amongst other marginalised social groups. In cultures where there seems to be less vitriolic hatred of fat people incidences of these diseases decline dramatically. Because of harassment, it is difficult for fat people to find non-judgemental healthcare, so we lose out on preventive healthcare, as well as medical attention when we are ill. Healthy lifestyles may be more difficult for fat people to accommodate into our lives than for thinner people. There are good reasons why exercise is off limits to fat people; the abuse, for example, that we get when we appear in public, or the unavailability of sports clothes in our size. We may also feel that there is little point in bothering to develop healthy lifestyles if we believe that as fat people we are impossibly gross and already beyond help.

Cultural beliefs about fat people interfere when we try to examine the real effects of fatness on our health. We have to cut away the myths which suggest that fat people are greedier and lazier than thinner people. In order to question the judgements made about us, fat people have to become adept at reading between the lines. We find that there is little consensus and that medical research is often contradictory in its evaluation of the health risks. The context of the research is also questionable. Scientific research trials, which inform most cultural beliefs about fat people's health, use samples of fat people who want to lose weight, rather than those of us who are comfortable with our bodies, or who no longer diet. In the US, trials have been advertised as free weight-loss programmes to encourage participants to come forward. These sample groups may have prolonged histories of dieting, and may suffer stress and dieting-related ill-health, as well as low self-esteem, yet this is rarely taken into account. Instead, it is assumed that the group is representative of all fat people, or that dieting and stress-related health problems are inevitable for us because we are fat. Furthermore, trials are initiated with hypotheses and general expectations for the results which may be weighted with assumptions. It is unlikely, for instance, that a trial which sets out to test a new weight-loss drug will find that the fat sample group are fine the way they are and don't really need this new product!

It could be suggested that fat women experience a double bind in terms of our bodies being classified as diseased. Later on I will discuss some of our interactions with health professionals, but for the moment let me say that within a medical and social context not only is our fatness seen as the problem, but as women our biological functioning is also regarded as suspect and as 'other' when compared to that of men. Medical science offers a way of dealing with this difference, hence the medicalisation of menopause as opposed to its celebration. Medical research is already a difficult area for fat people, but as AIDS activists have demonstrated, it is also an area where women are often marginalised, for example, through exclusion from samples in drug trials. If the predominantly female membership of fat rights organisations is significant, and if the assumption that it is mainly women who diet is a factor on which to focus, gender clearly *is* an issue for researchers investigating fatness. If researchers do not acknowledge this, there are negative implications for fat women's healthcare.

Fat people exist at a juncture where 'unhealthy' equals 'bad'. Our demands for rights and social acceptance are assumed to be invalidated by our unhealthiness, a condition for which we are responsible. Similar debates have occurred recently about the healthcare rights of smokers and substance abusers; that their care should not be a priority because they practise behaviour which is health threatening and that treatment provides a licence for them to continue; that healthcare should be withheld until they relinquish their 'bad habits'. But also that it is wrong for health workers to assume a moral authority which creates a hierarchy of 'good' and 'bad' patients, and no matter what the background, if someone is ill they need care. As fat people our ill-health is mostly assumed, we merely represent illness, but we are not immune to the health problems which affect everybody else. Usually our fat bodies bear little significance as to the way we experience an illness; however, because we want to challenge the myths about our assumed unhealthiness some of us try to play down our experiences when our fatness does affect our health. This need not be so. AIDS activists have shown that even when disease is associated with overwhelming prejudice and homophobia, sufferers have a legitimate claim on compassion, support, access to information, understanding, dignity, autonomy and social rights. I believe the same should be available for fat people.

Whilst I ally myself with the theories put forward by size rights advocates about the genetic roots of our fat bodies, and whilst I sympathise with their proponents, I question our need to find biological reasons for our fatness, especially singular explanations. If a whole movement of fat people hinges on one medical theory, what happens to us if that theory is successfully disproved or superseded at some point in the future? Would that invalidate our demands? The genetic theory is useful because it redefines our condition without the approbation of food theories, which project an element of choice on to our fatness. However, the genetic theory supports the notion that at least if we are not acting as villains towards our bodies, then we might be victims of them, that we 'just can't help it'. Disabled people struggling for rights often fight against being labelled as pitiful victims, which is a patronising definition that inhibits true social acceptance. I believe it is also inappropriate for fat people as a group of marginalised individuals to be labelled in this way.

To me, being fat is an identity more complex than the facts of my biological functioning or how my body metabolises food. Being fat is more to do with being socially marginalised, with finding out why we as a group are scapegoats, what that implies about social values, and how these beliefs and myths impact upon us all. I believe that basing our identities on medical theories confirms that we are in some way diseased, or rather an aberration from acceptable body norms, instead of being part of a wide spectrum of body types. The fact that there is so much interest in investigating our biology suggests that our difference is rooted deep within social attitudes – I have never read about any research into why so many people are thin, because thinner bodies are assumed to be the norm by which others are judged. Furthermore, I am sceptical about medical theories because I feel that whilst fat people are culturally reviled, biological explanations of our fatness will merely be used to support more complex attempts to make us lose weight, or prevent our existence in the first place. One day it may be possible to eliminate hereditary genes which carry a propensity for fatness, and if medical ethics still reflect the fatphobia in society, the medical establishment will condone this treatment.

Mental Illness

Fat people have been positioned as mentally ill largely because of a mixture of beliefs from traditional medicine and theories about eating disorders. The latter are now becoming contextualised amongst other mental illnesses such as depression, therefore since fat people are often assumed to be compulsive eaters, it is one small step further to assume that we are mentally ill. In theories exploring eating disorders, as we will see with the work of Susie Orbach and Kim Chernin, fat people are often excluded and marginalised as separate from the norm, as mysterious, frightening and dysfunctional. In addition to this, fat people have come to be labelled as mentally unstable in terms of traditional and popular psychological theories. It is assumed, for example, that we are addicted to food; that body size is an expression of inner conflict; that we were denied love as children and seek misdirected compensation by comfort eating. Freud's belief in the immature state of oral fixation seems to fit with modern beliefs that fat people are obsessed with food, especially 'childish' food such as cakes and sweeties.

Early fat rights groups were born out of the radical therapy movement on the West Coast of America during the late 1960s. This movement was critical of traditional psycho-therapy, which suggested that problems lay within the individual, and he or she should adjust in order to fit in with the rest of society. Instead, they asserted that people should not change in order to fit into an oppressive power structure, they believed that mental distress could be related to broad political injustices, and that changing oppressive situations collectively enables people to feel better as individuals. This position supports the idea that it is the systems in which we live that create mental distress. Some mental health activists, for example, have shown that black people are over-represented in the mental health system, and they suggest that this is an effect of racism. I know of no similar research specifically about fat people's experience of mental health, but I would suggest that, as with black people, it is not our cultural identities or our physical differences, such as skin tone or fatness, which cause many of us to feel depressed or agoraphobic; it is our dealings with a hostile culture, and our 'otherness' which make us vulnerable.

Although mental health campaigners have criticised this viewpoint, mental health is often believed to be congruent with notions of control, conformity and order. As fat people we represent what is supposedly out of control; instead of keeping in line, we have let ourselves go. When fatness is defined as a disease it promotes the notion that body size is a choice, if we do not make attempts to lose weight our motives also mark us out as suspect. After all, the dangers of obesity are well known, don't we want to be normal? Why not? As women our mental health may be affected by sexist standards of what is appropriate behaviour for us; for instance we may feel crushed by the social pressure to be passive or self-sacrificing. Similarly, fat women experience massive pressure to be slender, with terrible consequences promised if we fail to live up to this ideal. 'Self-respect' is often linked with stereotyped versions of how women should look, and since women's engagement with 'female diversions' such as beauty and dieting have often been a condition of recovery and rehabilitation, to refuse these activities puts us under suspicion. Orbach suggests that fat women reject patriarchal notions of femininity, and whilst I disagree with this blanket statement, it fits with the idea that we are categorised as 'crazy' because we are an affront to cultural values about feminine propriety.

Class

It has been well documented that class affects health; the more privileged a person is in terms of class, the better chance they'll have of good health. In comparison to disease, eating disorders and mental illness, class presents a more sociological explanation of fatness, where health is presented as a social rather than medical issue.

In stark contrast to the stereotype of the rich and selfish cigar-smoking fat capitalist, many fat people belong to the lowest socio-economic groups in Anglo-American culture, such as the poor, black, old or disabled. These groups are frequently misrepresented and misunderstood by more dominant classes, and beliefs have been generated about us that are offensive and which reinforce the notion that fat people are unhealthy. One example is that working-class people, as well as those of us who live in poverty, are fat because we are too ignorant to make healthy food choices. Another is that poor fat people overeat because we experience a collective unconscious memory of starvation, as in Stephen Mennell's rationale:

> It is hardly surprising if people drawn from the ranks of society where the fear for centuries had been simply getting enough to eat did not immediately develop self-control when suddenly confronted with plentiful food.[6]

This statement stereotypes fat people as primitives in a modern culture of plenty, who are lacking in self-control.

It implies that class is hereditary, held in one's body rather than externally constructed, and plays on the 'hopeless prole' attitude promoted by eugenicists. Richard Klein's discussion of class posits a patronising, almost Dickensian, view of working-class fat people.

> They pour their money into food and booze, and they find insulation in their fat against a scary world, where lack may at any moment brutally prevail. Their fat protects them against a cold wind, gives them bulk with which to feel stronger, and allows them to eliminate from their daily negotiations a great many desperate options.[7]

Another belief is that, as poor people, we can only afford cheaper food, which tends to be high in fat. This is a liberal argument which posits that poverty restricts one's choice of places in which to buy cheap and nutritious food. No matter how well-intentioned, I am wary of all these statements because they return to the tired equation that a fat body equals evidence of an inappropriate relationship with food, and that fat people are in some way responsible for the size of our bodies.

Class is an issue that is pertinent to fat people. According to Margaret Greaves, fat women are seven times more common in lower than higher socio-economic groups, which suggests that there are correlations between fatness and social, economic and cultural factors.[8] Why are there more poor fat women than rich ones? Especially since we are more likely to do physical work, and to rely on public transport, which negates the theory that we are fat because we lead sedentary lifestyles. Fat and class are also gendered issues; unlike women, lower-class men tend to be thinner than upper- or middle-class men.

There begs the question, does class status determine body size, or body size determine class status? Klein remarks that the statistical increase of fat people in the US coincided with the Reagan administration which brought rising levels of poverty. Greaves refers to *Social Factors in*

Obesity, a study from 1965, which found that fat women were less likely than thinner women to achieve higher social status than their parents, indeed it was more likely to be lower. This was not found to be true for men. Greaves also refers to H Canning and J Muir, *Obesity – Its Possible Effects on College Acceptance*, an American study which suggested that fat people were less likely to be accepted for college than thinner people with the same academic background.[9] Canning and Muir argued that this had implications for one's class status later in life.

Classist attitudes have prevented many useful explorations of why people of lower socio-economic groups tend to be fatter than other communities. This is an important area for discussion in terms of fat rights because it brings into question the idea that people can choose their body sizes. For example, although it is debatable whether people are able to choose their class background, the factors of age, race and disability are predetermined. A correlation between fat people and these groups could enable us to question the omnipresent medical definition of fatness, and to reassign it as a social issue rather than one of personal health.

Explanations

Explanations of fatness, whether in terms of disease, mental illness or class, and even size-friendly concepts such as set point theory, place our bodies within the world of scientific, academic and professional categorisation. Here, fat is something which must be dissected and resolved, it rarely exists in its own right, unlike, for example, slenderness. Explanations of fatness presume that our bodies are a problem or an issue, and imply a need for intervention.

Chapter Five
Eating Disorders and Red Herrings

Food and body shape are locked together in people's minds and eating disorders offer a popular interpretation of fat people. This is more a feminist than a medical debate, but it is one informed by health, and promoted by health professionals such as psychotherapists. In this context a fat body is considered evidence of, specifically, compulsive eating. Whatever our true experiences with food, this contends that fat people are fat because we ignore our body's natural hunger signals and eat compulsively, inappropriately. We eat in secret, and use food to deal with emotional difficulties. We have self-hating attitudes towards our bodies, which causes us to abuse ourselves with food. We try restrictive diets to enforce order upon our wayward bodies, but dieting itself feeds the cycle of denial and binge eating.

How have fat people come to be labelled compulsive eaters?

Whilst fatness is defined as a disease, or as abnormal, explanations will always be sought for its existence, and eating disorders seem to offer a diagnosis. Fatness is strongly associated with eating, despite growing acknowledgements that there are other factors in its genesis. The focus on disordered relationships to food seems to fit with general assumptions about fat people's eating habits. However,

> eating disorders are not really about eating; nor are they a 'slimmer's disease'. They represent the ways that some people find themselves using to cope with stress and other profound emotional or psychological problems. By focusing on food and eating, or not eating, they avoid facing those issues which they feel unable to resolve in any other way. The precise nature of the problem is different for each sufferer.[1]

Therefore, the motif of food and eating which connects fat people to compulsive eating may actually be quite tenuous. Indeed, recently eating disorders have been approached as a mental health issue.

In twentieth-century Anglo-American culture, many women consider their eating to be excessive or in need of control. Silence and shame about our true eating habits often prevents open discussion amongst women of what is normal. It is quite common for fat people, whose eating habits are already under suspicion, to identify as compulsive eaters in spite of our true eating patterns. Compulsive eating seems to offer a modern, progressive, medical, scientific, psychoanalytical explanation for what is often otherwise called 'greed'. Some fat people have grasped this label because it shifts responses to our bodies away from blame (that we're gluttonous and lazy) towards pity (that we're sick). We would rather be thought of as 'victims' of an illness than greedy 'villains'. I do not wish to deny that there are fat people who eat compulsively, but I also believe that there are many fat people who are inaccurately labelled as having eating disorders because we live in a culture which believes all fat people must have a disordered relationship to food. The repeated messages that fat people must be eating compulsively, or else we wouldn't be fat, also acts like a self-fulfilling prophecy. When such beliefs are reflected by authorities around us, even if they are inconsistent with our own experiences, it can encourage us to be concerned and obsessive about what we eat, and make us vulnerable to developing disordered eating patterns. In addition, underlying cultural values ensure that many behaviours associated with eating disorders, such as obsessing about body size, are regarded as normal for women. Consequently, since behaviour congruent with eating disorders is common, and trivialised as normal, many of us fail to identify what we do as harmful.

Another element of the debate around fat people and compulsive eating connects eating disorders to dieting. Eating disorders are regarded as an extreme form of dieting, although this view has been criticised, for example, by the Eating Disorders Association. Nevertheless, dieters and people with eating disorders play similar mental tricks on themselves in order to eat less and to lose weight, such as the denial of hunger, self-punishment and rule-setting. Since many fat people diet, we also display much of the behaviour of people with eating disorders.

Throughout common parlance, anorexia and 'obesity' are

positioned as opposites of each other – sufferers of anorexia are supposedly extremely thin because of a carefully planned strategy of not eating, whilst 'obese' people are very big because we eat too much, we eat compulsively. Such positioning places both groups within the context of eating disorders, but this is a false association. Eating disorders are behaviours, and although they can be characterised by weight changes, people of all sizes experience them, and many sufferers maintain 'normal' body weights. This contrasts with being fat, which is not a behaviour but a body shape. By polarising the two as opposites we create stereotypes, such as the image of the anorexic as bone-skinny or of the compulsive eater as fat – we cancel out the possibility of, for example, fat or 'normal'-sized people having anorexia, or thinner people suffering from compulsive eating. The association between anorexia and fatness encourages us to pitch one body size against the other. Since the majority of people are neither very thin nor very fat, these labels help distance both groups from the rest of society, and encourage people to ignore the implications that eating disorders or attitudes towards fatness might have for them. Indeed, fat people and those with eating disorders are presented to 'normal' people as freaks; it is assumed that our experiences have nothing to do with everyday values.

Feminists writing about eating disorders

The relationship between fat people and compulsive eating has also been reinforced by the influential legacy of feminists writing about eating disorders, especially Susie Orbach in her two *Fat is a Feminist Issue* books and Kim Chernin in *Womansize*.[2] Their work offered a critical means of examining women's relationship to body weight in a cultural context and popularised debates about the inefficacy of dieting, and the notion that fatness has a political significance.

These books are products of their times. Then, as now,

there was little documentation of the fat rights movement, and these works appeared to fill that gap, to offer new interpretations of the experience of being fat. They are part of the attempt to reclaim traditional patriarchal psycho-therapy and psychoanalytic symbolism on women's terms, and they owe a great deal to contemporary women's issues in Britain and America during the late 1970s, including the notion of the personal being political. They also draw on issues that are now regarded as troublesome with the feminism of that era, such as essentialism, psychobabble and the focus on white and middle-class women. In both Chernin's and Orbach's books the discourse is primarily about eating, not fat, but the distinctions between the two areas are blurred; 'fat' and 'compulsive eater' are often seemingly interchangeable in Orbach's work, and this is even reflected in the title, *Fat is a Feminist Issue*, not *Compulsive Eating is a Feminist Issue*. These books appealed to a very specific audience which happened to consist of predominantly middle-class and white women who had access to therapy and self-help groups in the 1970s. This audience included people familiar with feminist therapy principles, compulsive eaters and women with thinner bodies who said they felt fat as a way of expressing problems such as low self-esteem, as opposed to those whose physical reality was fat (although in *Fat is a Feminist Issue* both are taken to mean the same thing). Women who were members of these groups have testified that Chernin's and Orbach's work was very helpful to them. However, for anyone who does not come from the assumed readership, what at first appears straightforward in these books is confusing and complicated if read in a different context, for example, without the assumption that fat people have eating disorders, or without a knowledge of the language and values of psychotherapy. A lack of concrete definitions throughout these books leads to a lot of confusion; women describe their emotional outlook 'when I am fat' and 'when I am thin', but there is little distinction between who or what is fat.

These particular texts may be dated, and although they

were not initially intended as commentaries on fat people, the ideas they put forth continue to influence and connect fat people with compulsive eating. Despite their feminist intentions this is troublesome for fat women. Orbach's and Chernin's discussion of what it means to be fat is refracted through their perspective as thinner women with eating disorders, and this has led to some questionable assumptions being put forward.

Stereotypes

Orbach and Chernin promote stereotypes of fat women as anti-patriarchal rebels, victims and earth mothers. In *Fat is a Feminist Issue* Orbach suggests that the tensions women experience with our bodies are because we are oppressed as women. She argues that fatness is regarded as a failure in women since it implies that we are unable to control ourselves, especially our appetites. In a patriarchal society control is everything in order for women to gain approval by being submissive and 'feminine'. Therefore, by being fat, our bodies are a rebellious rejection of the pressures on women to look and act in limiting ways. But if being fat represents a mutiny against patriarchal culture, how does this explain those fat women who seek approval from men, who support and practise the rituals of a male-defined femininity, or who reject feminism? How does it address the dominant aspects of the size rights movement, many of which focus on the so-called 'feminine' pursuits of fashion and beauty? How does it reconcile fat women who court relationships as wives of Fat Admirers?

Initially Orbach defines fat people as cultural rebels, which could be flattering were it not for the stereotyped symbolism she imposes on fat women's bodies. The imagery of fatness is of a 'protective layer' around one's body, supposedly muffling our emotional responses to stress. The idea of a thin person imprisoned by a fat exterior is a cliché which will be familiar to anybody who has ever dieted, it reinforces the notion that one's body fat is something separate and alien from 'the real you'. Orbach uses psychoanalytic theory to embroider fatness with inherent and universal characteristics as though it had a life of its own, for example:

Fat *is* about protection, sex, nurturance, strength, boundaries, mothering, substance, assertion and rage.[3]

These labels are presumed to be objective and impartial but they are laden with Orbach's own values and subjective meanings. Only once in *Fat is a Feminist Issue* does Orbach suggest what she actually means by 'fat', when she describes women who weigh over 250lb as 'extremely large'.[4] In my experience of knowing fat women I would say this weight is on the smaller side of average. As I wrote in my introduction, defining who or what is fat is a tricky area, and I am uncomfortable with Orbach's blanket judgement; if she considers this size extreme, what is her take on larger fat women? It suggests that fatness is only acceptable up to a certain, smallish, point.

Chernin also attempts to find meaning in fat and thinner bodies, and the process of dieting. She asserts that anorexic women, and women who diet, are expressing a profound hatred and fear of their bodies, and have lost touch with the elemental female power which resides in the body fat of our bellies, thighs, hips and breasts.

Chernin proposes a limited vision of fatness: first, fat women are pathetic diseased victims, our bodies imply unacceptable eating habits and psychological disorder. In a passage referring to the novels of Margaret Attwood, Chernin speculates:

Taken together, these bear witness to the fact that the anorexic girl and the obese woman have a great deal in common. An unexpressed hostility, fear of sexuality, an uneasiness about what is expected of women in this culture, prompt both of them to take up their distinctive attitude towards food. Both are alienated from the body, and their natural power as women; both are, at least in the beginning, unable to express their emotional condition articulately and directly. Both use the body for the purposes of such expression. There is panic and self-hatred in both of them.[5]

Secondly, largeness in women conveys a socially inadmissable appetite for food, life and 'nurturant forces'.[6] Chernin invests heavily in the archetypes of the matriarch, primordial goddesses long forgotten who must be reawakened, and whose power women must reappropriate. Some fat women do choose to assume earth mother roles, but others (myself included), find labels like these offensive and clichéd when they are slapped on us by outsiders. The suggestion that fat women are powerful only occurs if we become symbols or comply with limiting roles.

Weight loss
Orbach and Chernin typify many feminists writing about eating disorders in that they are deeply critical of the Anglo-American cultural obsession with slenderness, but they have ambiguous attitudes to weight loss, especially for fat women. Orbach suggests that women try to find the underlying emotional reasons for their compulsive eating, and try to learn to eat for physiological rather than psychological hunger. This has since become classic advice given to people with eating disorders. However, in *Fat is a Feminist Issue* the advice is tempered with the promise that with a 'healthy' (ie non-emotional) attitude to food comes a body which has stabilised at an 'acceptable' weight. Orbach argues that we should rethink our attitudes towards acceptable body sizes, but to me 'acceptable' is a loaded term that really implies socially acceptable slenderness. Despite the assertions that it is the compulsive eating which is to be remedied, it is clear that weight loss is regarded as less of a pleasing side-effect (never alarming) and more of an overriding goal, as it states on the book's jacket blurb:

Throw away your diet sheets, stop starving yourself . . . and still lose weight.

In the introduction to *Fat is a Feminist Issue 2*, tiny statements hint at Orbach's attitude to fat people and weight loss. As part of a discussion of dieting she comments 'sadly we know that those methods work for very few people in the long run'.[7] Would she be happy if they did? Later she remarks that most people who diet regain weight 'and the ones who didn't need to reduce their size in the first place will live in the grip of anxiety around food and will be constantly watching themselves', unlike the fat ones who, it is implied, do need to lose weight.[8]

Culpability

Feminist theory around fatness and eating disorders makes many troublesome references to fat women 'making themselves fat', particularly as a kind of subconscious gesture against patriarchy. Being fat is initially perceived as an act of feminist heroism, but the implication remains that if we can choose to be fat we can also choose to be thin. Dealing with compulsive eating becomes just another way of losing weight. No matter how useful a weapon against patriarchy it is to be fat, keeping ourselves fat by compulsive eating has devastating emotional consequences, therefore dealing with our eating and stabilising at what will be invariably a lower weight is being more true to ourselves. This implies that truly healthy and functional women are not fat, at least not very fat; healthy women of an 'acceptable' weight are in touch with their bodies, their real and psychological hunger, but fat women are not; fat women are encouraged to 'give up' our fatness as though it were a bad habit. Feminist theory speculates that the 'original' part of us is thinner, and that our fatness is 'added on', and that fat acceptance is only a stage we must go through in order to achieve permanent weight loss. In *Womansize* Chernin also reiterates this, suggesting that we can choose the shape of our bodies through a new feminist aesthetic:

> according to health and nature, wishing our bodies to bear witness to our celebration of appetite, natural existence, and women's power.[9]

I question our ability to choose our body shapes, alongside the whole notion of one small group prescribing what is appropriate or 'natural' for women. The idea that individuals exert personal control over body size is central to traditional medical approaches to fat people, and theorists such as Orbach and Chernin also seem to reflect this. Although Orbach and Chernin promote self-acceptance in their work, the issue of exclusion (see below) suggests that fat women lie outside this possibility. They suggest that we are responsible for our fatness, that we have a free will, and if we don't like our bodies it is up to us to do something about it. There is an underlying drive towards personal change, revitalising and reinventing ourselves in the pursuit of happiness, rather than accommodating self-acceptance or seeking social change. This individualistic solution sits uneasily with the social context in which these theorists place their debates. *Fat is a Feminist Issue* and *Womansize* have enabled thinner women to question traditional medical theories about their behaviour, whilst reiterating them for those of us who are fat. Finding parallels between women's struggles with weight and women's wider social disadvantages is useful and helps us politicise 'personal' issues. Paradoxically, by identifying fat women as compulsive eaters, and therefore dysfunctional, these writers *de*politicise our fat bodies by medicalising us.

Exclusion
Ironically, despite references to 'fat' and 'size', fat women are excluded from Orbach's and Chernin's texts, both covertly, by unacknowledged prejudice, and explicitly. For

example, *Fat is a Feminist Issue* is not about fat people, and Chernin writes expansively about the meaning of fatness, fat women's power, our psychology, but comments:

> Granted, I say, there are obese people in this country. But I am concerned here with the large numbers of us who think we are overweight when we are not and spend the better part of every waking moment pursued by a nagging worry about the pseudo-obesity we suffer from.[10]

I do not 'suffer' from 'pseudo-obesity', my fat is real. By releasing this disclaimer Chernin positions fat women as 'other' and eliminates us from a thesis which purports to define our identities and lives.

The legacy

Feminist analyses of eating disorders that were new and radical in the 1970s now seem familiar and acceptable to most people with an interest in body issues. Whilst they have cleared the way for a deeper understanding of the effects of eating disorders, they have also largely defined many of our 'progressive' attitudes towards fat people as 'other', mysterious and disordered. Consequently, we are stuck with an anachronism which prevents us from growing and developing our ideas about what it is to be fat women.

Today, Orbach and Chernin seem to have steered away completely from their association with fat rights issues. This is not surprising as such a discourse was never intended to be a primary focus of their original work. Their more recent books are more clearly defined as addressing anorexia,[11] and mother–daughter relationships,[12] and there is less of the confusion overlapping debates about fatness and eating disorders. However, their earlier work continues to influence people writing about fat.

Fat is a Feminist Issue is used as a model of recovery in books by Jo Ind and Irene O'Garden,[13] two compulsive eaters who identify at various points as fat. Naomi Wolf, like

Orbach and Chernin, discusses fat women within the context of hunger, and eating disorders; of thinner dieting women who think they are fat. In a piece about black women and recovery, bell hooks supports the notion that fat women are disordered and dysfunctional by discussing fatness in the context of food addiction (as she terms compulsive eating). hooks argues that because black cultures have a more accepting attitude to fat women it is very easy to hide food addiction.[14] This statement presumes that fat women are fat because we are food addicts or compulsive eaters in the first place. Writing about lesbians, Valerie Mason-John also contextualises fat as a food/eating issue, discussing anorexia, bulimia and compulsive eating seamlessly alongside personal case studies which include an anorexic woman, a bulimia sufferer and several fat women who do not explicitly identify as having eating disorders.[15] Susan Powter appears to make a feminist criticism of dieting, attacking diet industries, asserting that dieting is detrimental to women, only to offer a low-fat diet plan of her own.[16] This fits with Orbach's ambiguous attachment of weight loss to recovery within a context that is critical of the culture which supports dieting. The suggestion that fat people should 'make peace with food' to stabilise at an 'acceptable' weight, and the notion that body size is controllable also runs through Klein's musings on fatness, and he, like Wolf, continues the practice of labelling women's fatness and thinness with inherent meanings: fat represents rebellion, fecundity, whilst slenderness connotes obedience. Other writers, such as R M Meadow and L Weiss[17] include fat women who do not identify as having eating disorders and references to fat rights initiatives in discourses which are primarily about eating disorders. Using fat women and organisations as positive role models may be a useful strategy to encourage a readership to acknowledge that fat hatred is not inevitable. However, because this is not explicit, the inclusion of fat people in these pieces continues to imply that, regardless of our experiences with food, we are central to debates about eating disorders.

Fat Women and Eating Disorders

Interestingly, writers who have come to address fat people without the filter of eating disorder theory have largely ignored those discourses. Margaret Greaves recognises the implication in *Fat is a Feminist Issue* that fat women have eating disorders – she is critical of this, but agrees with other aspects of Orbach's work, that body fat operates as a protective desexualising layer. Sue Dyson also refutes the claim that fat people habitually suffer from eating disorders, although she uses some of Orbach's exercises from *Fat is a Feminist Issue 2* in her chapter on recovery and self-esteem.[18] Shelley Bovey disregards the suggestion that fat people are compulsive eaters, but discusses her anger and discomfort with anorexics because they appear to have rejected fatness so violently.[19] Carol Wiley includes material concerning fat women who have experienced compulsive eating but this is presented as case studies, and there is no critical commentary which might explain their context and surrounding debates.[20]

To my mind the connection between fat people and compulsive eating is complicated; obviously some fat women are sufferers, but the response to this, and the more general assumption that all fat people have a dysfunctional relationship to food, is unsatisfactory. Whilst writers and practitioners who come from an eating disorder perspective marginalise and stereotype fat people, the response amongst fat writers has been inconclusive. Is the issue too complex or thorny to address?

Meanwhile there are real consequences both for fat and thin people. If we are anorexic, bulimic or a compulsive eater, the misinformation about fat people and eating disorders can affect the treatment that sufferers of all sizes can expect to receive. For fat people, recovery is often attached to weight loss, whilst the continuing devaluation of fat bodies can be devastating for people who have kept their natural weight low through self-starvation or vomiting, and who are frightened of gaining weight.

Equally worrying is when a fat person is misdiagnosed as having an eating disorder. If the person is not a sufferer it can leave them feeling alienated and confused; if they are, and the disorder has not been identified, it might worsen and the sufferer could miss the help and support that are needed.

Chapter Six
Cures

Conceptualising fatness as a health problem carries the corresponding assumption that somehow it must be cured. Even genetic explanations of fatness, so popular with fat activists, can be interpreted in this way, which is one reason why genetic engineering is such a threat to us; are we going to be wiped out? In the meantime, for fat people the 'cure' is inevitably weight loss. Humans are believed to be accountable for the size of our bodies, so changing our body shape and losing weight is regarded as an attainable option. An element of choice has crept in, and with choice comes duty. Losing weight 'for the sake of one's health' is lauded as a responsible gesture.

Losing weight, even through illness, is often assumed to be therapeutic, and this is especially true for fat people. Suggestions that we try to lose weight are amongst the first instructions that health professionals issue when we are ill and when we seek help for health-related issues, such as infertility. Indeed, treatment that is standard for thinner people, for example, certain operations or drugs, may be withheld from us unless we lose weight. In this chapter I discuss and criticise some of the most common methods by which fat people are encouraged to lose weight within the context of the medicalisation of our bodies, and then I offer a different paradigm.

Weight-Loss Treatments

Dieting

As we have already seen, in terms of losing weight, fat bodies are explained by the basic model which asserts that there is more food energy going into our bodies than we can use. We store this energy as fat. Fat is unhealthy and unaesthetic, therefore the solution involves restricting the amount of food energy that enters the body in order to use up fat and restore the body to its lean ideal. There appear to be many ways of losing weight, but almost all of them rely on this equation, and generally, weight-loss schemes translate into practising various dietary constraints, including the amount and type of food we eat, such as its calorific or fat value. We go on 'diets' which may be short- or long-term and take many forms from liquid fasting, eating meal replacement biscuits and milkshakes, to low-fat 'healthy eating' regimes. Sometimes we follow diets from books and women's magazines; more often we impose our own personal restrictions, such as eating only salad or processed diet food.

Alongside dieting there are other methods which restrict

the amount of food energy that enters our bodies. 'Behaviour modification' refers to the mental tricks we utilise in order to eat less; eating only between certain times of the day, using small plates to make the amount of food on them seem larger, wearing an unremovable cord around our waists which cuts into us uncomfortably if we put on weight, using the best crockery and glassware to make eating seem like a special occasion, eating very small amounts of sweets as a 'reward' and so on. Other methods include exercising to 'burn up' calories and fat, vomiting, swallowing laxatives or taking appetite suppressants. Max Airborne says:

I've also done more secret things, like getting ill and not taking proper care of myself in the hope that I might lose weight, or just plain starving myself by not eating anything for days.

Dieting, by itself or more often combined with behaviour modification, is the most familiar and widespread option people take for losing weight. Fat or not, most women diet in some form and at some point in our lives, and in Anglo-American society it is considered part of women's culture to do so.

The mythology that surrounds dieting implies that it is good for us, that it works, and that it will make us feel better. But over the past thirty years, women's criticisms of dieting culture have gained momentum. Feminist academics and cultural analysts, women involved with therapy and self-help groups, women coming together in other organisations, or accessing information from fat rights groups or the media, have begun to question the role and effects of dieting on women. Typically, what fat people have been saying for years, the evidence we have gleaned from our own experiences, has only recently been acknowledged and bolstered by findings from various scientific research communities, who have an interest in finding out the effects of dieting, and why it doesn't work.

They feel that research in this area could lead to breakthroughs in finding a weight-loss method that *does* work. A breakthrough is potentially very lucrative, and many researchers are supported by commercial diet companies, as well as traditional medical fundholders. I am not suggesting that all scientists researching the failure and effects of diets are so avaricious; many have an altruistic interest in health issues and fat rights. However, I would argue that we examine the context from which criticisms of dieting are made in order to place them within the wider field of size rights activism.

In the short term a closely followed reducing diet will cause a person to lose weight. However, fat rights advocates suggest that dieting interferes with one's set point (see p 11), and therefore the rate at which our system metabolises the food we eat. Dieting convinces our bodies that we are starving, so after the initial rush of lost weight our metabolisms slow down in order to protect our reserves and survive on less. Many dieting organisations have 'maintenance diets', or suggest that dieters change their eating habits 'for ever' because when one stops dieting, one's body protects against further periods of starvation by storing more food energy as fat, so that the more 'successful' a diet is the higher the chances of regaining weight. Moreover, 95–98 per cent of people who diet inevitably regain not only the weight they lost on that diet, but frequently more, according to a study in 1992 by an American organisation, the National Institutes of Health.[1] Dieters find that dieting increases their weight and Klein suggests that fatness may be an 'iatric disease', which is one caused and exacerbated by health and beauty professionals, all of whom promote dieting and weight loss.[2]

Earlier in this book, the interview sample commented on how dreadful diets made them feel, and during my discussion of the health risks of being fat I mentioned how people who repeatedly lose and gain weight are at risk of developing or aggravating heart disease. There are other illnesses connected to dieting. In 1994 the Body Image Task Force, based in California, started producing a label listing illnesses connected to dieting based on research by Janet Polivy and Peter Herman of the Psychology Department of the University of Toronto, as well as information from fat rights commentators. The label was used by women as part of a campaign to discredit dieting industries. It was pasted on to diet products in shops, on reply-paid coupons for diet clubs and in diet books. It reads:

> WARNING: Dieting has been shown to lead to anxiety, depression, lethargy, lowered self-esteem, decreased attention span, weakness, high blood pressure, hair loss, gall bladder disease, gall-stones, heart diseases, ulcers, constipation, anaemia, dry skin, rashes, dizziness, reduced sex drive, menstrual irregularities, amenorrhea, gout, infertility, kidney stones, numbness in the legs, weight gain, eating disorders, reduced resistance to infection, lowered exercise tolerance, electrolyte imbalance, bone loss, osteoporosis and death.

Weight-loss diets do not necessarily indicate a healthy diet. Since companies such as Nutri/System were sued in 1990 by people in the US who experienced gall-stones and health problems after following their programme, many members of the industry have backpedalled over the sale and use of diet aids, such as meal replacement milkshakes and biscuit bars, which can be very high in fat. Even diets that appear 'healthy' can be too low in fat, or too high in processed food, additives and chemicals. All diets for weight loss short-change our bodies in one way or another.

Dieting is psychologically questionable. Diets are addictive, and encourage individuals to play the same emotional tricks on themselves as do people with eating disorders. When we diet, we might find ourselves becoming obsessive about food, feeling frightened and insecure about what we eat, ignoring our body's natural hunger signals, or rubbishing our self-esteem. Although sticking to a diet is demanding, dieting seems to offer a solution that appears to satisfy some of our deepest yearnings. The desire to transform our bodies, for example, can be very powerful. Transformation offers hope for new beginnings; it is magical, and it overrides everyday problems. But diets don't fulfil their promises, and there are better ways of improving one's life through realistic, permanent and attainable goals.

Sometimes we are in situations that are beyond our control and a new diet offers us the chance to feel that we are 'doing something about it'. This is contradictory, since dieting entails relinquishing responsibility for one's life by following a set of regulations. They help us to ignore other problems, but fail to address the underlying issues. Mary Evans Young comments that one of the benefits of dieting is that 'it's a known entity, therefore safe and sound'.[3] The familiarity of dieting rules and rituals can be a comfort, can help us cope, and rules offer validation and support, which might otherwise be lacking. In an uncertain world rules suggest certainty and predictability. But it is a false security and is based on suppressing our true feelings in order to fit in and make other people feel comfortable. Furthermore, when the diet has inevitably failed to produce permanent weight loss, perhaps because of the inability of a person to sustain a lifestyle based on denial and sacrifice, and when a dieter experiences all the problems that are part and parcel of dieting, it is the dieter who feels that they have failed, and never the institution of dieting that is questioned. Wolf refers to the cult-like methods used by diet groups: they foster an unchallengeable authoritarianism where conformity and belief in the process is prized and deviation punished; they encourage individuals to sacrifice their current 'unhealthy' social connections in order to experience a kind of spiritual renewal; and they promote a kind of moral superiority: 'We have the answer'.

The businesses that promote weight loss have so far been

very lucky in selling people a pretence of authority. A lack of regulation, and what seems to be a remarkable immunity to advertising standards legislation, has put dieting industries in a very profitable position with no need to be accountable to anybody. Dieting is big business, dieting products are expensive and profit margins are high. The industry depends on formulating new ways of selling us the myth of weight loss, of manipulating our desire, in order to part us from our cash, so the market is saturated with 'gimmicky' weight-loss products: 'fat-dissolving' cream (often accompanied by the phrase 'to be used in conjunction with a calorie-counted diet'), or 'fat-burning' vitamin pills, or body wraps; the permutations are endless. These depend more on fashion and popular culture than the scientific model mentioned earlier – for example, when nicotine patches for smokers first appeared in the early 1990s, they grabbed the popular imagination to the extent that a 'diet patch' was also launched! The industry does not care for us, it is interested only in overstating the dangers of being fat and playing down the health risks of dieting so that it can string us along as happy consumers. Bizarrely, although they are marketed with the promise of success, dieting products cannot be too effective, because if dieting really worked there would be no diet industry, and no profits, as there would be no unattainable dream to sell.

Dieting is a crossover issue that fat people share with others of all sizes. Campaigns, articles in the media, and organisations which criticise dieting offer a good platform on which a whole range of women can come together. However, there is rarely an acknowledgement of how the experience of dieting can be different for women of varying sizes. We are caught in a catch-22; we know that diets cause many problems, but fat people continue to receive the mixed message from a variety of sources that weight loss is always assumed to be beneficial for us. Critics of dieting have tended to ignore, marginalise or stereotype fat people in their arguments. My friend Elaine Smith, a fat woman and artist, comments:

There's been a couple of things on quite recently and although they've said 'don't diet because it can be quite harmful for you', then they've almost turned it around and said, 'You don't want to be too much over – a few pounds is all right, there's no point in worrying about a few pounds.' So they're not really talking about really fat, they're not talking about stones overweight, they're talking about a few pounds overweight, so it's no good worrying over three pounds. They're not really talking about allowing people to be any size. I always think it's quite conflicting; on the one hand you think, 'ooh! People are actually coming round to the idea that dieting isn't good', but then they sling that in and you're still 'oh well, this doesn't apply to me'.[4]

Many critics still cling to the notion that although dieting is undesirable, it is preferable to being fatter than a certain kind of 'moderate' fatness. This position sets up divisions between 'good', ie smaller, and 'bad' types of fat people and implies that criticisms of dieting industries do not apply to all fat women.

Drug therapy

Weight-loss tablets and 'food supplements' are sold in healthfood shops, by pyramid selling companies such as Herbalife (those people who wear LOSE WEIGHT NOW, ASK ME HOW badges), and in the backs of magazines. In this section I do not intend to discuss these types of drugs since they are widely derided by medical practitioners. Instead I mean to review drugs based on, or acting like, amphetamines which have the effect of suppressing one's appetite.

Diet pills can be bought over the counter in the US, but in Britain they are not so freely available. In the past they were often prescribed to women of all sizes who expressed an interest in losing weight. Nowadays thinner women tend to be discouraged from taking them, due to an increased awareness of dependency risks and eating disorders. Like all amphetamines there are significant and detrimental side-effects, including dependency, insomnia, paranoia and heart disease. However, they continue to be offered to fat women. In 1996 the British government sought more controls over the prescription of these drugs based on evidence that they had been implicated in the deaths of at least fifteen women. Despite these deaths, there was no call for a total ban on slimming pills because they are still believed to be a useful aid to 'the clinically obese'. It would seem we are expendable.

Drug therapy seems to offer a quick fix for fat people: it is comparatively cheap, easily administered and does not entail the dramatic lifestyle changes that other weight-loss methods demand. These reasons can also be drawbacks; women have a long history of being overlooked by health professionals and pushed into treatments which are convenient for others, but which do not necessarily suit us. With drug therapy, women are vulnerable to being prescribed for long-term use drugs which can seriously damage our health. Sometimes we are complicit; as a culture we have much faith in the superiority of medical science over other kinds of action, and we are tempted by the prospect of a tiny 'magic pill' which appears to be able to transform us painlessly into thin people, and which could solve all our problems.

Could a miracle weight-loss pill exist? All medicinal drugs come with side-effects and even those rare drugs which have transformed medical history, like penicillin, at their most magical have only the power to alter one small (but important) part of the illness. In modern medicine, miracle pills do not appear from thin air; they have a chemical history, they are researched, and they are conceived for profit. The idea of a 'miracle pill' is a potent one, and one that other marginalised groups have considered. For example, some black activists during the 1960s talked about whether they would take a pill, if it existed, to make them white. Thirty years on the notion that it is desirable for black people to become white or that a continuing struggle for civil rights could be reduced to the issue of whether or not to take a pill is offensive. More recently, the search for a miracle drug that cures AIDS is underway, with many charities sponsoring research. However, some AIDS activists are widening the debate to ask questions about the politics of drug-manufacturing companies, about who would profit from such a drug, and about potential hazardous side-effects. Fat activists take note.

Like a new diet, the notion of a miracle weight-loss pill is mostly a fantasy, and far away from the reality of taking a drug. However, the search is on to expand the number of weight-loss drugs on the market, particularly in the US where the Food and Drug Administration are seeking to 'fast-track' trials of weight-loss drugs. Fast-tracking stems from the US government's attempt to 'do something' about what they define as the problem of obesity in America. This has culminated in a government-sponsored programme, the National Institutes for Health's 'Shape Up America' initiative. Fast-tracking would reduce the amount of time spent on tests that are mandatory for licensing, and enable companies to launch new drugs on to the market more quickly. Dexfenfluramine is one weight-loss drug that has been fast-tracked in the US and is now available there on prescription as Redux. It is chemically related to amphetamines, Ecstasy and fenfluramine. The last of these is another diet drug whose use has been associated with brain damage and memory loss. In addition, users of dexfenfluramine may experience diarrhorea, nausea and an increased risk of heart disease, after which dexfenfluramine tends to produce only a small weight loss in its takers. Fast-tracking drugs works in favour of drug companies who want as many of their products out on the market as quickly as possible. The increase in weight-loss drugs available, and the willingness to prescribe them before proper trials in order to 'Shape Up America', suggests profits and politics are being put before fat people's health.

Psychiatry, psychotherapy and counselling

Where fat is defined as a mental illness, or a symptom of deeper psychological problems, psychiatry, psychotherapy and counselling are used as methods of promoting weight loss, the idea being that once the internal struggle is resolved, so is the 'weight problem'. Whether or not the desire for weight loss is a primary goal, or more covertly implied, when fat people enter therapy there are some issues to consider. There are many different kinds of therapeutic talking relationships, and a myriad theoretical backbones to support them. Some are client-centred, others work against a backdrop of established philosophical or ideological systems. Although therapy and counselling are health professions, they are not always conducted by medically trained workers.

Of the more medical styles of therapy, traditional psychiatry is not always user-friendly and mental health activists have been very critical of its potential to disempower clients. Unlike counselling and psychotherapy, which are more often available to middle-class people, or those who are able to pay, and where boundaries are clear and more equal, psychiatry is available to everybody in Britain free on the National Health Service. Sometimes people are coerced into psychiatry against their wishes, and psychiatrists have the authority to prescribe drugs and various treatments, and to overrule a person's consent. I am concerned that since many fat people are of low social status we are at risk, when we seek help, of becoming channelled through the psychiatric system, disempowered and labelled 'mad'.

Given that feminist therapy was instrumental in developing issues around eating disorders where fat people were defined as compulsive eaters, which contributed to the classification of fatness as a mental illness, it is unsurprising that talking cures for weight loss have become popular. Many of us make contact with a psychiatrist, a therapist or a counsellor with the prime intention of losing weight and sometimes this desire is encouraged by them without any discussion of the context from which it came. In the backs of magazines, on community noticeboards, some therapists advertise themselves as experts in dealing with 'weight problems', or by offering 'dietary advice'. Counselling as a profession is considerably unregulated and open to various interpretations. Weight Watchers' group leaders, for instance, call themselves counsellors, cashing in on the trust, status and implied impartiality that surrounds the role. Therapies can tend towards gimmicky treatments which, like all methods of losing weight, rely more on fashion and a user's fantasy than any quantifiable results.

Most of us enter therapy to deal with a wide range of concerns, many of which are unconnected to body size, but where some fat issues arise. Therapy can help us challenge these areas and feel happier or more fulfilled. Having space to talk about our fatness can be wonderfully liberating if the practitioner is sensitive and able to listen without judgement. We may find that our problems will not be solved by losing weight. But sometimes weight loss is covertly implied as a health-enhancing strategy, regardless of whether or not this is true. If the main reason for therapy is to promote weight loss, any progress is seen only in that context and therefore can only help the individual develop a partial understanding of what it means to be fat. It is also a judgemental agenda, which does not accept fat people as valid. Clients in therapy make themselves vulnerable, even suggestible. Fat people in therapy must be careful that we do not automatically take on the values of the practitioner, particularly if they harbour fatphobic attitudes.

Surgery

I do not intend to discuss liposuction, abdominoplasty or lipectomy, which literally remove areas of fat, as these operations tend to be performed on thinner women to reduce the size and shape of specific body areas. For fat people there are different kinds of fat-reducing surgery which take effect by reducing the amount of food that can be taken in by one's body.

Surgeons have been developing weight-loss surgery since the 1950s, when the first jejuno-ileal (small intestine) bypass was performed. There are several types of intestinal bypass operation but all basically entail the surgical shortening of one's intestines, which prevents food being absorbed into one's body, creates constant diarrhorea, and enables the body to lose a large amount of weight quickly. For the patients whose post-operative state is rated 'excellent' (approximately 40 per cent), normal side-effects include dehydration, electrolyte imbalance, malnutrition, cirrhosis, metabolic and psychiatric problems. Long-term complications include an increased risk of kidney stones, enteritis of the severed intestine and liver failure.[5] Often patients must undergo more operations. According to Ernsberger and Haskew:

> Intestinal bypass was the first surgical weight-loss procedure to achieve widespread routine use, and remains the most effective means of long-term weight reduction, since regain is slight as long as four years postoperatively. Unfortunately, intestinal bypass is also the most dangerous weight-loss method, over 28 separate complications have been identified. Death rates of 4 per cent to 6 per cent are common.[6]

In a private communication Ernsberger remarked that these death rates are only short-term figures and that the ultimate death rate is higher in the long run. He asserted that in most cases the operation must be undone eventually because 'it is incompatible with life over the very long term'.

Intestinal bypass operations have decreased in popularity, not because of the high death rates involved but because they have been eclipsed by other less risky procedures. Jaw wiring physically stops a person from eating solid food for a time period from a month to a year, although it does not prevent anyone from liquidising whatever they want to eat. It is a 'public humiliation' method of weight loss, since it is awkward to carry on a normal life when one cannot speak because one's jaws are wired together, and consequently one's visibility enables other people to police one's food intake. People who have their jaws wired together are encouraged to carry wire cutters with them, since there is a real danger that they could choke to death should they vomit. Two less popular surgeries are oesophogal banding which prevents a person from swallowing, and the gastric balloon, a device which is inserted into a person's stomach to create a 'full up' feeling and inhibit the amount of food they can eat. Unfortunately the balloons tend to break. All of these procedures have found limited success and high rates of weight regain. But despite its problems weight-loss surgery is profitable, especially in the US where most of these procedures originate, and more interventions are being developed.

One surgical development which has increased vastly in popularity over recent years is stomach stapling, a term that includes several different types of operation which share a similar outcome. Stomach stapling is performed on fat people considered by their doctors to be at least 100 per cent fatter than their 'ideal body weight' according to height and weight charts. Under a general anaesthetic a surgeon places a plastic band around the neck of one's stomach which acts like a sphincter muscle and reduces the amount of food that can enter. The size and shape of a person's stomach is then physically reduced by a stapling mechanism, which limits one's stomach capacity for food drastically. Because a person's stomach cannot then accommodate much food, weight loss is inevitable, although dieting must still be maintained. Stomach stapling is not as perilous as previous weight-loss operations, but it is still *very* risky. It involves major surgical intervention and starvation. A stomach staple is intended to last for ever, but bands and staples break frequently, patients can find themselves facing several repeat operations and experiencing the same attendant risks.

Weight-loss surgery appears as a breakthrough for fat people. After surgery we believe that we can eat what we want, albeit in smaller amounts, and still lose weight; our bodies have been modified to take care of everything. Surgery transforms fat people relatively quickly into individuals who look 'normal' and can live normal lives free from fatphobic harassment, which makes it very attractive to people who may have suffered years of abuse and self-hatred. But a staple does not solve every problem. The individual must continue to diet, anything more than the smallest portion of food is vomited, and some people who have had this surgery report that they 'cheated' and became obsessed with finding ways of eating 'forbidden' foods, such as liquidising chocolate bars. Some people regain the weight lost. Nevertheless, the price of impairment, pain and major health complications, perhaps for the rest of your life, and sometimes even death, is still considered a fair exchange for a tenuous slenderness.

With the desire to lose weight so strong that we will risk our lives for it, it is questionable that we are able to make an informed decision to undergo the operation. Ideally we should be able to find clear and objective information about the risks and benefits of the procedure, but this will be unlikely when the health professionals who offer these procedures are themselves steeped in fatphobic beliefs and cultures, not to mention the surgeons eager for guinea pigs on whom to try new techniques. Few fat people in Britain have access to groups such as NAAFA's Weight Loss Surgery Survivors' Special Interest Group, where more realistic information about living with the effects of such surgery can be shared. Objectivity and thorough explanations may be impossible when weight loss is positioned as such a desirable goal by patient, doctor, surgeon and the surrounding culture. Surgery is seductive.

In my heart, I felt the operation was a coward's way out. It really meant that someone else was doing for me what I didn't have the will-power to do for myself. But I was so desperate, I agreed straight away.[7]

Pre- and post-operative counselling may be minimal, and with so much at stake, a patient may be unwilling to consider any alternatives:

In today's climate it is naive to expect most patients to show regard for their own health, so over-riding is their desire for weight loss. This issue has become particularly clear in the experience gained with weight-loss surgeries. Many surgical candidates show a striking lack of interest in the risks. After surgery, they ignore severe and unpleasant side-effects rather than allow the procedure to be undone. 'Our female patients', write Ravitch and Brolin (1979 pp382–391), 'have been reluctant to accept the dismantling procedure, even when it was discussed in terms of saving their lives.'[8]

The irony of weight-loss surgery is that it is performed on *healthy* fat people, but it destroys rather than enhances our health. A further irony is that in other areas surgeons often refuse us non-fat-related surgery and anaesthesia until we lose weight, saying our weight makes surgery dangerous, but these same risks don't seem to apply when the reason for the operation is to make us thinner.

The major health risks associated with weight-loss surgery seriously outweigh the advantages of increased self-esteem, which could also be gained by cheaper, no-risk, non-surgical means. These surgeries also support a system of fat hatred. Yet many fat people want this operation and surgeons are willing to deliver the service. This has led to a sense of complacency surrounding weight-loss surgery; it is performed mainly on people who are very fat by Anglo-American cultural standards and is considered to be an effective way of dealing with us. After suffering years of self-hatred, surgery seems to offer a final solution, but no attempt is made to understand why we should feel so negative about ourselves in the first place, nor are there efforts to find safer alternatives.

Self-help

Self-help weight-loss groups fall into two categories: non-commercial and commercial. The former can include informal groups of friends who diet together, groups where weight loss for fat people can be part of the wider aims of therapeutic organisations, such as Overeaters Anonymous, as well as activity groups, such as exercise classes run by local authorities. Commercial groups include organisations like Weight Watchers, or those instigated by magazines, and personalities such as Rosemary Conley.

Non-commercial self-help weight-loss groups exist to enable women to come together for mutual support, to overcome isolation and loneliness, and for fun and social contact. Groups can be as informal as friends or colleagues meeting regularly as a diet club. Having access to support is cited by diet proponents as an important factor in getting people to lose weight. However, there can be many problems with groups such as this. Groups can be places where negative beliefs about fat people and fatness germinate, and therefore self-hatred is surreptitiously encouraged and excacerbated by the pressure of a number of people believing the same thing. Groups may have little knowledge of some of the issues around dieting, and they can be fertile places for the development of eating disorders if sufferers go unchecked. In therapy-style groups there may be less chance of members resolving problems in their lives if exploring one's feelings is considered merely an adjunct towards losing weight. People caught between conflicting group dynamics can find themselves unable to speak out for fear of condemnation or of losing friends. Friendships can also become ruined by the rivalry of weight-loss competitions.

Some non-commercial groups, such as Overeaters

Anonymous, have been likened to religious cults. Overeaters Anonymous is related to various addiction support groups such as Alcoholics Anonymous and Gamblers Anonymous. It is a support network which runs groups for sufferers of compulsive eating. Women turn to the group when they are particularly vulnerable and are encouraged to follow the famous Twelve Step Programme to recovery. Critics are concerned that there are no regulations concerning groups like Overeaters Anonymous, that they can teach what they like, and that members become very dependent and evangelical about them. My concern is that Overeaters Anonymous bases its recovery programme on stereotyped beliefs, similar to those outlined in *Fat is a Feminist Issue*, about what one's fatness is 'saying', and about fatness indicating pathology and disorder.

Some non-commercial gatherings do not advertise themselves specifically as weight-loss groups, but losing weight is the main reason that women attend. For example, local authority leisure centres provide exercise classes with titles like 'Fatbusters' and 'Over Forties Fatties'. Groups like these, where activities are performed primarily for weight loss, can provide an outlet for compulsive exercisers, a focus for body hatred, and because the shared desire to lose weight is unspoken, there is less chance of group members ever questioning it.

Commercial diet groups can find their history in organisations such as the Women's League for Health and Beauty, founded in Britain in the 1930s. The League was the first to offer 'keep fit' classes to working-class women in village halls and factories. Women had previously been excluded from sport and physical activity because it was considered unladylike. By associating exercise, diet and hygiene with the more socially acceptable realms of beauty and femininity, the League hoped to improve women's health. Commercial weight-loss groups continue to meet in local community centres, schools and church halls. Women who are isolated in their communities can find friendship and camaraderie in these groups, since an important role of weight-loss groups is to bring women together for mutual support. However, the actual ethics of weight loss and the source of the social pressure to lose weight are never called into question.

Despite the cosiness of the environment, profit is the bottom line in commercial weight-loss groups. The weekly membership fee does not amount to much, but it adds up as members work through the cycle of losing weight, regaining and rejoining the group over periods of years. Commercial self-help diet groups operate as franchise businesses, like McDonald's and Coca-Cola. Under various conditions, for a fee and continuing royalties, individuals can buy the right to use the company name. In most cases, employees originally approach the parent company as clients. As they become more involved, they buy a franchise, become 'self-employed' group leaders, and run local groups. In this way the parent company is able to expand and increase profits for a minimal outlay of finances and resources.

Commercial groups also use many familiar but lucrative marketing strategies, such as offering a range of products, including drinks and ready meals, that group members are expected to buy; or having tie-ins with other services and products – one year, for example, Weight Watchers offered free membership to consumers of Special K diet breakfast cereal. Companies also sponsor weight-loss competitions and hold slimmer-of-the-year publicity extravaganzas where the famous 'Before' and 'After' photographs are always in evidence. They target advertising campaigns in the new year and at the beginning of the summer when people are likely to feel insecure about their bodies, and they follow the tradition of buying celebrity endorsements. In the past, famous fat people such as Cyril Smith MP and the astrologer Russell Grant were approached to represent companies by losing weight on their diet. But even fat celebrities inevitably regain the weight they lose, which is embarrassing for the diet businesses. Nowadays thinner personalities, such as the actress Lynn Redgrave, are promoted since there is less chance of them yo-yo-ing so dramatically.

Self-help weight-loss groups combine conflicting ideologies through their form and content. These groups have roots in the feminist tradition of women coming together and sharing experiences to effect a deeper understanding of ourselves and the politics of our lives, but they can be authoritarian, conservative, restrictive and more concerned with profit than with women's health. I am not opposed to businesses making money *per se*; what is distasteful is that commercial self-help weight-loss groups profit from services which don't fulfil their promises, by perpetuating myths and stereotyped ideas about how dreadful and unhealthy it is to be fat. In doing this they are disempowering their clients rather than helping them. They market themselves as community groups and are never upfront about their profit motive. They promote a system of authority and deference: leadership as opposed to collective action, rewards for weight loss and punishment by shame when there is no loss. These groups embody deeply conservative values, where the preservation of authority and the status quo is paramount and not to be challenged, and for women who take part in such groups, the traditional sexist bindings of femininity (such as being thin and pretty in order to catch and keep a man) are promoted as an asset, not a liability.

Is it worth it?

Weight-loss treatments are basically ineffectual, and compromise rather than enhance our health. Fat people are encouraged to lose weight by any means possible, even if there is a real risk that it might kill us. When fat people die from trying to lose weight, the cause of our death is invisible; it is always our fatness that is blamed. Where some treatments are regarded as successful, success is ambivalent; for example for a diet to 'work' one must starve on it for the rest of one's life, and effective weight-loss surgery at its 'best' produces numerous dangerous side-effects. Despite these shortcomings there is little expectation amongst many fat people that there could be any other choice; the only solution to the problems we deal with is of being cured of our obesity disease, so we allow ourselves to be guinea pigs for the latest scams. Losing weight means that we can take our place in normal society; it makes us feel acceptable. When we lose weight we experience the euphoria of fitting in – it is an addictive feeling of having succeeded, but one that is inevitably short-lived.

In order to be healthy and functional, fat people do not need to lose weight. Health depends on many factors, some of which are stress management, adequate housing and warmth, love and respect, a balanced diet, physical activity, mental well-being and good self-esteem, all of which can be attained at any size. Fat people are part of a spectrum of body types, all of which have positive and negative health attributes. Fatness is normal. Whilst we are surrounded with negative messages about the inherent unhealthiness of fatness it is impossible to distinguish what the true risk factors might be, likewise the health benefits. But no matter what these risks are, the hazards inherent in weight loss will not make us well. The notion of a cure for fat people shares parallels with various Victorian gynaecological theories which regarded women as inherently ill and abnormal compared to men, and where brutal medical treatments, such as clitoridectomies, were conducted in order to 'cure' what was already normal, healthy and natural. Modern-day attempts to 'cure' normal healthy fat bodies through weight-loss treatments are equally futile.

Medicalisation

Medicalisation is the process by which various social groups are defined purely in terms of their biology and anatomy by medical professionals in order that they can categorise and understand them. It is the medical naming of 'unusual' phenomena ('unusual' only according to narrowly defined norms) as something that is sick and in need of curing. Members of what we might now call social groups have been medicalised in the past: black people were believed to have smaller brains than white people, women's sexual and reproductive organs were thought to direct women's behaviour, homosexuality is still regarded in some environments as a disease, and disabled people continue to fight medical labels. The erroneous medical categorisation of social groups has had terrible consequences: stereotyped beliefs based on medicalisation inform much of what is racist, sexist, homophobic and disablist today.

Medicalisation is problematic because it establishes norms by which people can be measured. Normality is always considered the most desirable status. Where people do not fit these norms they are classified as abnormal and invalid; for example, disabled as opposed to able-bodied, or gay as opposed to straight, fat as opposed to thin. Aside from setting up false polarities, as there is no acknowledgement of the grey area in between these classifications, it is arrogant to measure people who represent a wealth of diversity against one standard from one dominant culture; it enforces a patronising value judgement on the quality of our lives.

Medicalisation characterises a deep faith in science in twentieth-century Anglo-American society. Science is held as the zenith of knowledge; it orders the chaotic world into a logical framework and deals with events through universal laws and abstract concepts. It deals with facts unsullied by human emotion. Medical science has dramatically transformed modern lives 'for the common good'; we no longer die from diseases which decimated earlier generations, and it is therefore regarded as progressive and its practitioners as trustworthy.

Medicalisation treats social issues as medical issues. Social issues have political roots, they are affected by such interventions as legislation, changes in attitude and social trends, whereas medical science is believed to be 'factual', unbiased and unaffected by such things. Of course this is untrue; medicine is as much affected by fashion and opinions as any other discipline. Indeed, Ernsberger and Haskew remark that dieting as a medical therapy originated because of the influence of dieting as a fashionable pastime in the 1920s and 1930s in Europe and America.[9] Science is not apolitical; its proponents live in the same cultures as everybody else, they deal with the same problems, they share interests and prejudices, and are not immune to human nature. Politics is as much a part of medicine as in other areas of life, even party politics, as recent cuts to the National Health Service in Britain demonstrate. The founding fathers of modern medicine, as well as the majority of practitioners today are members of an exclusive group, not only by virtue of their education, but also through their social class, gender and ethnic background. They reflect the dominant culture's values, and have power and status enough to construct their knowledge as superior and legitimate.

The cultural faith in medical science and its practitioners has led to fat people's reliance on professional health experts. Professionals have an interest in supporting medical definitions of fatness, and sometimes medicalisation, because their values, status and livelihood depend upon it. Hence, with the medicalisation of fat people, the health risks of being fat, and our dependence on health professionals to 'fix' us are exaggerated whilst the risks of losing weight are underplayed. This is partly because professionals usually have an active role to play when we undertake weight-loss cures, but are generally absent if we strive for self-acceptance or personal empowerment. Experts are educated, they have a knowledge of health issues, and sometimes the power to prescribe treatments for us. Both for the lay person and the health professional there is an expectation of paternalism; experts are authority figures who we hope will 'take care of us' when we are vulnerable. However, a doctor–patient relationship where the doctor is in charge fosters passivity and dependence. This can cause problems since many health professionals harbour negative attitudes towards fat people. Wooley notes that many doctors regard fat people as 'weak-willed, ugly and awkward' and 'self-indulgent', and health professionals 'who were most knowledgeable about obesity were as negative as others towards the obese'.[10]

As fat women, our expectations of health professionals contrasts dramatically with our experience of them. Fatness is generally regarded as the root of whatever problem we may be suffering from. Kristine Kay sums up: 'If you go with an ingrowing toenail, it's "because you are fat".' In twentieth-century Anglo-American culture and medicine, fat people are understood to be responsible for our size, and health professionals often make rude, patronising and unacceptable comments about our bodies. Communication can become very strained and charged with anxiety. Yvette Williams Elliott was on the receiving end of comments by her GP that made her feel dreadful:

> I went home and howled, and I would often come home from the doctors and throw up . . . I haven't actually been to the doctor's now for five years, and I've had a few things wrong during that time which I felt I really ought to have done, to have seen someone, but I haven't. I'm too frightened to.[11]

Health professionals present weight loss as the universal panacea for fat people, in spite of the known risks, and harangue us into various weight-loss schemes. This can become a substitute for real healthcare. When we complain or demur, many health professionals regard it as a challenge to their authority, not a chance to learn something new; they pull rank and react with disbelief or ridicule. Whether or not we accept or reject the inevitable admonishments to lose weight, this strategy can leave us feeling invalidated and undermined at a time when we are most vulnerable and in need of help. I never go to see my doctor; my illness or discomfort must be massive before I will even contemplate arranging an appointment. As a fat woman I must evaluate my need for healthcare against the censure, rudeness and inappropriate treatment I am liable to be offered when I present myself to health professionals. Because of this, I often fear that my health is at risk.

The medicalisation of fat people works to mystify our bodies. Where medicalisation establishes norms of thinness, we are encouraged to feel abnormal, ashamed and desperate. We turn to health professionals for help but find the cures on offer to be questionable, whilst other options, like self-acceptance, are never discussed. Moreover, the medical explanations which define us as pathological and the useless treatments we suffer are politically convenient. This means we constantly blame ourselves when weight loss inevitably fails, not the context that pressurises us to become thin. When we do begin to demand rights, the misunderstandings medicalisation has engendered for fat people, for example, that we have eating disorders, has set a precedent for yet more red herrings.

A Social Model

Medicalisation ensures it is the fat on our bodies that is blamed for the problems with which we deal. Fat-hating beliefs insist that it is our bodies which are at fault, that losing weight is a choice we should exercise in order to adapt and fit in. However, disabled people offer an important theoretical precedent for challenging this assumption. These debates are rooted in earlier civil rights and feminist struggles to reframe 'the problem' in a social context, and whilst not wishing to negate their contribution, I have decided to focus on disability rights as a paradigm because it is a contemporary model which explores how cultures deal with bodily difference, it supports a new social movement and, to me, these reasons are what makes it most appropriate and relevant to fat people.

The 'social model' redefines disability as less of a problem of one's physical difference compared to able-bodied people, and more as a phenomenon created by cultural attitudes. For example, traditional and medicalised beliefs suggest a disabled person might be disabled because they have one leg instead of two. In the social model, this kind of difference is called an impairment, there is no comparison to able-bodied people, it is just another bodily variation. Disability instead refers to the social attitudes and cultural or physical barriers which prevent people with a variety of impairments from playing a full part in everyday life. Disability is redefined, so disabled people are not disabled because they cannot walk; a wheelchair user with a mobility impairment is disabled by buildings which do not have ramps; a person with a sight impairment is disabled by books which are not available as a tape recording or in braille; other people are disabled by attitudes which prevent them from becoming one's friend, one's employee, or one's lover.

A social model enables us to regard our bodies not as abnormal or shameful, but as part of an infinite spectrum of body types. Redefining fatness in a social context enables fat people to challenge the disempowering authority of medicalisation, as well as other fatphobic institutions. As with other social theories, the social model demonstrates that aspects of our personal lives have a significance in the wider environment, and that certain events we experience as fat people are a result of social attitudes, instead of our personal shortcomings. Moreover, the social model encourages us to stop feeling as though our fat bodies are the cause of all our problems, and helps us to refocus our energy on to the social contexts and attitudes which endow us with such low status. For example, we don't have to blame ourselves for being too fat when a seat is too narrow, instead we can direct our anger towards the disabling beliefs that seats do not need to be very large because bodies only come in a few limited sizes.

With the social model it is society which needs to adapt and change to meet our needs, not vice versa. This model offers us support as we are now. It is an empowering paradigm, not a patronising one, and using it as a way to understand our oppression can enable us to cultivate a more positive identity, both individually and as a social group.

Are fat people disabled?

Identifying ourselves as fat people as 'impaired' and 'disabled' requires sensitivity. One disabled friend argues that impaired is too charged a label for fat people, since it implies to her the physical ill-health, disease and low medical status from which fat people are struggling to distance ourselves. I have no such problems with 'impaired'; I regard it without a value judgement. There is an uneasy sense that by appropriating the label 'disabled', fat people are invading and colonising the achievements of disabled people. But this implies that the social model is 'their' work, something which belongs to 'them', not 'us'. It implies ownership and relevance to only one section of society, rather than a theory which is more universally liberating. Perhaps there are other labels and identities for fat people which need to be uncovered or reclaimed.

Fat and disabled people experience many things in common, and perhaps this will predispose us to be more understanding and accommodating of one another. However, like most of us, disabled people live in cultures which harbour fat-hating attitudes and are not immune from internalising such values. Some disabled people might also resent fat people identifying as disabled if fatness is believed to be self-inflicted, and therefore less legitimate than an impairment which is not regarded as such.

If fat individuals begin to publicly identify as disabled, not only do they risk rejection from disabled people, but also from communities closer to home. The social model of disability is unfamiliar to most able-bodied people, and their attitude towards disabled people is often pitying, fearful or awed by the 'tragic but brave super-crip' stereotype. Fat people are no exception and I suspect many of us would refute the label 'disabled'. Whilst able-bodied and disabled people are culturally and institutionally segregated it becomes difficult to build a positive or realistic image of what it is to be disabled. In size rights communities I sense a palpable fear of disability, and attempts to constrain disabled people as separate. For example, in a discussion of early fat rights groups in the US, Judy Freespirit recalls:

> Back then NAAFA's [National Association to Advance Fat Acceptance] tack on 'civil rights' for fat people was to do volunteer work for the Cerebral Palsy Association to show fat people were nice.[12]

Karen W Stimson points out that fat activists cannot afford to harbour such patronising and misinformed attitudes towards disabled people and disability.[13] In the US since the late 1980s numerous discrimination cases have been won by fat people where their fatness was defined as a disability and they were therefore protected under federal disability laws. These laws offer rare legislative protection for fat people's civil rights. We would be foolish to let our prejudice interfere with real chances for justice and equality.

Fat Health

I believe in a person's right to control their own body, even if that entails putting it through something that I would not choose myself, such as weight-loss surgery or simply another diet. Unfortunately, the more we realise how bogus many of the findings of scientific research and medical attitudes are, the more difficult it becomes for us to make informed choices about our health. We find that there is very little non-judgemental information available to us, and rarer still are the health professionals who can empower us with fat-sensitive facts. Because medical research and beliefs are skewed against us we cannot make objective declarations about whether being fat does indeed damage one's health. We have lived with the assumption that it does with appalling consequences, and now we are beginning a different experiment. With precedents such as the social model of disability, fat people are trying to redefine ourselves as healthy and normal, learning not to judge our thrilling diversity as one biological entity, and acknowledging that even if our fatness does compromise our health by putting us at risk for various diseases, we deserve the same care and attention as anyone else. Losing weight is not an option because it *does* damage our health, and if we are indeed found to be susceptible to disease, we will need to preserve as much energy and vitality as we can.

The debate surrounding whether fat people are healthier or less healthy than thinner people is inconclusive and works as a smokescreen preventing us from demanding our rights:

> Given that permanent weight loss is elusive for most fat people, the issue of fat and health is irrelevant. The only true option available is to be as healthy as you can, regardless of your weight.[14]

Whilst health and medicine are separated from politics, we find it very difficult to think of our struggles as having political significance because our medicalisation as fat people suggests that it is we who are invalid, we who must conform, and we who must take responsibility for becoming 'normal'. I think we also fail to consider that health is a cultural construction, and that what is acceptable in one context is not in another. This is not to say that health is not an issue for fat people. We need access to non-judgemental healthcare that will increase our well-being and respect our bodies, not 'cures' which punish us for being fat or put our health at risk. We need an end to medical bullying, and an increase in health professionals' sensitivity towards us. We must acknowledge that although fatness itself is not a disease, that doesn't mean we shouldn't revise our cultural values about how we relate to disease and illness, which are presently very demeaning to people who live with disease. In the end, it is society that needs to change, not us.

Section Three

The Fat Rights Movement

Chapter Seven
Fat Rights History

The social model of disability offers fat people one way of framing fat hatred. However, fat people are a diverse group and span all social strata; we need not one but a whole range of theories to match our complexity. Over the past three decades a movement of fat people has been evolving which encompasses an enormous variety of perspectives and ideas. Like disability politics, this movement seeks not to 'rehabilitate' fat individuals to shrink into 'normal-sized' society, but to effect a fundamental change in cultural attitudes towards fat people. This chapter charts the history of some key organisations and individuals who have influenced this movement, first in America and more recently in Britain. It is a brief overview that looks at size rights on a national rather than a local level since there is very little documentation of the smaller support groups which may have existed at the time.

American Fat Rights

NAAFA and the Fat Underground are not the only size rights initiatives to have emerged in America, but they were the first, and their work paved the way for many aspects of the movement today, such as the involvement of professionals, the proliferation of support groups and the explosion of consumer goods and services, all of which I will go on to discuss later in this book.

NAAFA

As with all political movements, the Fat Rights Movement started with dissent at grass roots level. It was not until 1969 that the first recognised organisation was established. NAAFA, formerly the National Association to Aid Fat Americans, now the National Association to Advance Fat Acceptance, is the grandparent of the fat rights movement, and is regarded by many as a blueprint organisation. It was established in 1969 by William Fabrey, who was angry about the discrimination suffered by his fat wife Joyce. He became influenced by the work of Llewellyn Louderback, author of *Fat Power*, who criticised dieting and argued that American society is prejudiced against fat people.[1] Fabrey envisioned a group of fat people and thinner supporters who could develop Louderback's ideas and fight size discrimination.

Fabrey started NAAFA as a group campaigning for civil rights, since Louderback had already placed fat people alongside other civil rights struggles of that time, such as early feminism, gay liberation and black power. These were grass roots movements generated by the people most affected by the issues. Surprisingly, NAAFA was not founded by a fat person – Fabrey himself was not fat at that time yet he considered himself an appropriate person to start the group. During an interview, he recalls:

> When I began NAAFA, all the fat people I knew had bought into the prevailing myth that said they were inferior because of the size of their bodies. It took me – a thin man, someone not in their oppressed group – to have enough self-confidence to fight for size acceptance.[2]

For many years NAAFA's roots in civil rights movements were eclipsed by its more lucrative and popular social function, which still flourishes today. The group created services which would encourage new people to join, such as large-size fashion shows, parties and workshops; it provided places for people to socialise, including dating and pen-pal programmes; it provided information through leaflets and the NAAFA book service; and members could find support through local chapters.

Over nearly thirty years the organisation has taken on a more multifaceted appearance. Based in California, NAAFA now defines itself as a non-profit human rights organisation 'dedicated to improving the quality of life for fat people by means of public education, advocacy, and member support'.[3] It publicises information on legislative issues and new research findings through a newsletter. NAAFA's Fat Activist Task Force organises protests and letter-writing campaigns to fight size discrimination, successfully challenging, for example, Hallmark Greetings Cards who then withdrew a series of cards featuring offensive comments about fat people. NAAFA has more than fifty volunteer local chapters throughout the US, and there are national conventions and special events, as well as regional gatherings. NAAFA convenes a variety of special interest groups (SIGs), which produce their own newsletters and activities. These include: the Big Men's Forum, the Feminist Caucus, the Lavender SIG for lesbian, gay and bisexual fat people, and the Lesbian Fat Activist Network; groups for couples and single people; groups concerned with health issues pertinent to fat people such as diabetes and sleep apnoea, a Mental Health Professionals' SIG and the Weight Loss Surgery Survivors' SIG; groups for families and young people including the Parents and Caregivers of Fat Children SIG, Teen/Youth SIG, and the Young Adult SIG; groups for fat people of various sizes, including the Super SIG, and the Mid-Size SIG; there is even a group for people with a special interest in military issues.

NAAFA is the largest size rights organisation, and widely respected. This is not to say that it does not have its critics. Karen W Stimson explains:

> In the mid- to late 70s I was a chapter member of NAAFA and very active at the local and national level. I was on the National Board of Directors and served as Chapters Coordinator, my earliest networking activism, as I tried to help new chapters and established ones stay alive with virtually no support from NAAFA – whenever I'd ask, 'What is NAAFA doing for its chapters?' I'd get the answer: 'NAAFA exists'. It was a frustrating job but it did put me in touch with the Fat Underground, which was on NAAFA's shit list after the former Los Angeles chapter seceded. I was one of a handful of East Coast NAAFA fat feminists, which made me a lot of enemies among the NAAFA hierarchy.

In autumn 1995 a group of NAAFA National Board members publicly resigned amidst recriminations and much anger over the organisation's use of resources. In February 1996 the board of directors voted to become self-perpetuating rather than be elected by ordinary members. Some grass roots members are feeling increasingly disillusioned and disenfranchised by this development, they are discouraged with national NAAFA's management. Meanwhile local chapters continue to flourish and attitudes towards them are still very positive. Based on her experience in New Mexico, Karen Smith comments:

> While working with our local chapter has been a blessing, the National naafa continues to be an embarrassment and a millstone around our necks. One thing I don't think naafa fully grasps, is that it is no longer the only game in town. I feel that local grassroots impacts of our organization are the most valuable work of fat acceptance . . . the only way you can change is one person at a time. And we can do that whether our name is New Mexico naafa, or whether our name is the New Mexico Largely Positive Group, or the New Mexico Fat Acceptance Assn. At the present time, there are very few benefits of remaining affiliated with the name naafa, since the present leadership obviously has no feeling for the discontent rampant in the chapters and continues to dwell in its ivory tower.4

As a result of their disillusionment with national naafa, groups such as the one Karen Smith belongs to have now begun to secede from the parent organisation, and a new network of fat rights initiatives has germinated.

The Fat Underground
The current conflicts within NAAFA are not unique. During the early 1970s the Fat Underground formed partly out of a dissatisfaction with the parent organisation.

The Fat Underground began with Aldebaran, later known as Vivian Mayer, a fat woman with a 15-year history of dieting. She and another fat woman, Judy Freespirit, were members of the Radical Feminist Therapy Collective in Los Angeles. Radical therapy attempts to find political connections to 'personal' problems, in order to empower individuals to seek collective change. In 1972, impressed by Louderback's *Fat Power*, Aldebaran and Freespirit discussed his ideas within the context of their feminism and radical therapy.[5]

During 1973 Aldebaran and Freespirit became members of the Los Angeles chapter of NAAFA. Aldebaran expressed many misgivings about its structure, for example, she found a lack of communication between her local chapter and the national organisation. There were also political differences; at that time NAAFA did not support the increasing confrontation between fat activists and health professionals. Aldebaran and Freespirit, who were grounded in radical lesbian and feminist politics, grew dissatisfied with NAAFA's conservative perspective. In a letter from 1974, Aldebaran states:

> It is clear to me now that my support for NAAFA is not for *all* NAAFA activities – for example, I oppose the computer dating service, the emphasis on how fat people also can be happily locked into nuclear families, fat women as sex symbols – I oppose them politically and understand, I think fully and compassionately, their appeal for fat women and men who are at a more conventional place politically. I don't want to help fat men obtain privileges [sic] that will set them clearly over me.[6]

The Los Angeles chapter then left NAAFA with some members forming the Fat Underground. Later that year Aldebaran and Freespirit wrote the Fat Liberation Manifesto, which allied fat oppression with the struggles of other oppressed groups, criticised dieting and diet-supported industries, and called for equality, respect and civil rights for fat people.

The following year, 1974, marked an explosion of activity for the Fat Underground. They published Position Papers defining fat oppression in connection with sexism, job discrimination, an inaccessible public environment, health issues, stereotyping (particularly in humour and comedy), health professional's detrimental attitudes towards fat people especially in psychiatry and food issues.

The Fat Underground staged showdowns with health professionals and diet clubs. Lynn Mabel-Lois (now Lynn McAfee of the Council for Size and Weight Discrimination) advised members to use medical libraries to discover the real research results for themselves. What the group uncovered formed the basis of subsequent arguments about fat people and health, debates and discourses mentioned in earlier chapters which are now central to fat politics.

The Los Angeles Radical Feminist Therapy Collective had a problem-solving group, many of whose members joined the Fat Underground to form consciousness raising, support and their own Fat Women's problem-solving groups. Members of the Fat Underground also brought a new awareness of fat rights issues into the community by representing fat people in coalitions, and networking with other groups and individuals.

The Fat Underground demonstrated against unfair and inaccurate representations of fat people in the media. After Mama Cass, a singer with The Mamas and Papas, died from a heart attack that was certainly exacerbated by strenuous dieting, it was reported that she had choked to death on a ham sandwich. The Fat Underground were outraged by this distortion of the truth and held a public demonstration at the Los Angeles Women's Equality Day. Aldebaran writes:

On August 25th, in the middle of the celebration, Lynn Mabel-Lois of the F.U. went on stage and gave a speech eulogizing Cass and indicting the medical profession for her murder. Cass Elliot starved to death – the medical profession has studied reducing diets long enough to know how deadly they are. At least twenty fat women walked up on stage with Lynn, carrying candles and raising clenched fists. Some of them were strangers who joined the march on the spot, as soon as they heard what Lynn was going to say. I was surprised at how wide the feeling and consciousness has reached.[7]

As well as criticising the media, the Fat Underground used it to distribute information about fat politics. They contributed articles to newspapers, magazines and newsletters, as well as publishing their own pamphlets. Later, Fat Liberator Publications distributed packets of leaflets and photocopies of important articles.

In the mid-70s personal differences amongst Los Angeles radical feminists caused splits the community, and several Fat Underground members left Los Angeles. On the East Coast Aldebaran, Sharon Bas Hannah, Karen W Stimson and Stimson's then husband Darryl Scott-Jones formed the New Haven Fat Liberation Front. They carried on working in the style of the Fat Underground, debating, holding workshops, producing articles and spreading the word. In Los Angeles, the Fat Underground continued for a short while, and then disintegrated.

The Fat Underground may have been very specifically of their time and location, but they left a powerful legacy for subsequent fat activists by introducing their feminist politics to fat people's experiences. William Fabrey comments:

> The first people to use words like 'oppressed minority' when referring to fat people were the women involved in the Fat Underground in Los Angeles in the early Seventies. The collective writings of these radical feminists, which later were published in *Shadow on a Tightrope*, did a lot to sensitise the rest of us to the oppressive components of our struggle.[8]

The Fat Underground was innovative because it was formed by and for fat women, and its analysis of fat people was borne out of direct personal experience. Furthermore, the research conducted by the Fat Underground around fatness and health became an influential resource for sympathetic health professionals. Two famous papers, *Obesity and Women I – A Closer Look at the Facts* and *Obesity and Women II – A Neglected Feminist Topic*, by psychologists Susan C Wooley and Orland W Wooley drew much of their information from the Fat Underground, making the ideas palatable enough for other professionals to draw inspiration and follow suit.

Although the Fat Underground did not survive as an organisation, Stimson explains that in the 1980s different generations of fat feminists in the US developed the ideas it sparked.[9] She talks about a fat women's community that became visible through articles in feminist magazines, such as *Off Our Backs*, *Sojourner*, *Matrix* and *Sinister Wisdom*, through support and activist groups, and through conferences and workshops. Between 1980 and 1982 FAT (Fat Activists Together), a coalition of fat feminists, developed *Shadow on a Tightrope*. This book grew out of the past decade's fat feminist community, including work from members of the Fat Underground, pieces from Fat Liberator Publications, material from workshops, as well as personal and theoretical contributions. Towards the end of the decade fat feminism gained recognition from the National Organisation of Women and *Ms* magazine, two powerful and prominent US organisations. Women's publishers began to address the issues and, furthermore, NAAFA finally acknowledged the feminists' contribution through Board membership and the NAAFA Feminist Caucus.

The British Contingent

The fat rights movement is even younger in Britain. For a long time debates about the politics of size were sealed within feminist discourses around eating disorders and looksism. For example, Nancy Roberts, who presented the *Nancy at Large* and *Large as Life* series for Thames Television, published *Breaking All the Rules: Looking Good and Feeling Great No Matter What Your Size* in 1985. This book mixes autobiography with Orbach-esque material, and Roberts discusses coming to terms with compulsive eating through her work with the performance group Spare Tyre. Much of *Breaking All the Rules* consists of Roberts' fashion ideas, with case studies of other fat women, who are also featured as models. As a reader of this book, Currey says:

> It was the first time I had seen images representing fat women as attractive, and often with great individual style. It shows a wide cross-section of female imagery, from glitter and power-dressing to dungarees and cotton smocks, and with hairstyles, jewellery, scarves etc to strengthen the looks being shown. This book was enormously liberating to me in terms of starting me on the path of accepting my size. It also helped me overcome my strong inhibitions about getting pleasure from a fat body, through having fun with things like clothing.[10]

As I have pointed out earlier in this book, contextualising fatness within debates about eating disorders can be problematic, and it has only been since the late 1980s, when British fat people began to find out about the growth of NAAFA and fat-positive initiatives in the US, that the politics of size began to be examined in its own right by the magazine *Extra Special*, the Fat Women's Group, and in Shelley Bovey's book, *Being Fat is not a Sin*.

Extra Special

Perhaps excited by the success of mainstream plus-size fashion magazines in the US, such as *BBW*, clothes retailer Eleanor Graham published *Extra Special* independently between 1986 and October 1988. Fleetway then acquired the title and it was promptly discontinued. *Extra Special* took the form of a women's weekly magazine, it was available from local newsagents and had the usual articles on beauty, knitting, recipes and fashion. Unlike other magazines it purposefully marketed a positive image of fat women, and included articles such as 'The Right to be Large', whilst using large-sized models, and featuring interviews with fat celebrities. *Extra Special* also had regular keep fit, medical advice and agony columns specifically for fat women.

Many of *Extra Special*'s angles were innovative – there had never been a mass-produced, popular magazine which featured and celebrated fat women in Britain before – but some aspects of its philosophy were confused, such as the notion described in one of Graham's editorials that obesity and largeness were different, that a 'large lady' was not necessarily obese, and that only obese people should diet and lose weight. This was a divisive message; *Extra Special* often printed material suggesting the pointlessness of dieting, and now it seemed to be distancing itself from the fatter members of its readership. The magazine's avoidance of the word fat, using endless references to 'larger ladies' and 'big girls' was also a source of irritation for some people. However, *Extra Special* was radical for its time, and Yvette Williams Elliott remarks:

> *Extra Special* was quite important in that I was buying it and it coincided with my decision to stop dieting so it felt political just to buy it. I think although it was very fashion focused from what I remember, that in itself was an important first step for me. I wouldn't say it was enough, but it was a start.[11]

Extra Special also set the pace for other British women's magazines to follow, such as *Pretty Big* and *Yes!*.

The Fat Women's Group

The original London Fat Women's Group began in 1987, with some meetings between fat women who wanted to address fat oppression. Tina Jenkins explained in 1988:

> I read *Shadow on a Tightrope* about three years ago and that was the first time I'd come across these sorts of ideas. A woman who'd also read the book and wanted me to write an article for *Spare Rib* phoned me up. A few of us met for about a year.[12]

The group's ideas evolved into a big feature in the feminist magazine *Spare Rib* in 1988. The group wanted British feminists to deal with fat oppression and the politics of appearance, and over several pages Tina Jenkins and Heather Smith explained some of the basic principles of fat oppression and fat feminism; Barbara Burford provided a personal account of being fat; and the piece ended with a list of supportive resources. Afterwards many women wrote in response, and the London Fat Women's Group was created as a fat feminist support and activist organisation which aimed to develop a national network of similar groups.

In 1989 the London Fat Women's Group convened the National Fat Women's Conference. With the first sniff of publicity the British media pounced. Group members appeared on popular television programmes such as the *Wogan* chat show, as well as more sophisticated slots like *Open Space*, with its public access format. This provided a huge audience for the ideas of this small feminist group and rocketed fat issues into people's lives. The publicity created additional problems: the conference became vastly oversubscribed, media coverage was frequently tokenistic and hostile, the organisers had to eject journalists in attendance in order to create a safe space for the participants, reporters harassed delegates outside the conference building, whilst the paparazzi attempted to take secret photographs of a dance workshop.

The conference was an empowering day for most of the delegates. The opportunity to trade shared experiences was especially validating, and the day was the first chance for many women to discuss fat issues. Organiser Heather Smith remarked 'It was great to see so many of us move centre stage'.[13] The conference was based on a programme of workshops dealing with health, sexuality, employment, clothing, drama and dance, plus additional groups exclusively for lesbians, black and working-class women. Workshop participants wanted to form ongoing special interest groups, for example to lobby the NHS to provide

non-judgemental healthcare for fat people. Recommendations for the future direction of fat issues were presented
during the plenary, for example, some fat women wanted
to build coalitions with other groups. The conference was
intended for fat women only, and instead of dictating a
range of admissible body sizes, one of the underlying
principles was self-definition. Consequently thinner
women attended who identified as fat, which some people
found difficult.

In the months after the conference, the London Fat
Women's Group experienced burn-out and in-fighting.
Many of the debates that were splitting the wider feminist
movement, for example, around class and sexuality, were
also being played out within the group, there were also
personal differences. The London Fat Women's Group
eventually disintegrated.

I could not attend the conference, but in 1989 the
London Fat Women's Group made a big impression on me
whilst I was beginning to develop ideas about my identity
as a fat woman. I moved to London in 1990 and, not
knowing that the group no longer existed, tried to find
them. During my search I made contact with other people
who were interested in fat liberation. By 1992 I realised
that there was no Fat Women's Group, so I decided to
restart it. Although I resurrected the Fat Women's Group,
I am no longer involved. The focus of the current group is
changing; as well as being a support group and producing a
newsletter, *Fat News*, in November 1996 members
curated an exhibition entitled *Positive Images of Fat
Women*, and in 1997 organisers Diana Pollard and Tracey
Jannaway launched SIZE, a new campaigning group.

Being Fat is not a Sin

In *Being Fat is not a Sin* Shelley Bovey developed an
understanding of fat oppression which eclipsed both *Fat is
a Feminist Issue* and *Breaking All the Rules*. *Being Fat is
not a Sin* was the first British book to discuss fat people in
terms of discrimination and civil rights. Bovey explained

that prejudice against fat people permeates many aspects of our lives, especially in medicine, and historical and cross-cultural accounts demonstrate that beliefs about fat people being unhealthy and ugly are a twentieth-century Anglo-American phenomenon. Bovey criticises the fashion and dieting industries and the way they support fat hatred, and *Being Fat is not a Sin* describes how being fat influences our self-image and our closest personal relationships. By the time *Being Fat is not a Sin* was updated and retitled *The Forbidden Body* in 1994, many of Bovey's observations were in common currency.

Bovey refuses to mouth simplistic platitudes about fat people. Many fat rights advocates are eager to present an image of fat people as beautiful, capable, smart and exciting. No wonder, when most representations of fat people portray us as stupid and ugly drudges. Although she does not clearly define whom she means, Bovey deplores what she names the 'Big is Beautiful Brigade', a group of people I take to be those smiling, somewhat sanitised fat women featured in magazine make-overs and throughout the mainstream media whenever size issues surface. Bovey says:

> This only further isolates fat people, making them another category by the use of positive discrimination. It is the apologist's approach. Big is Beautiful does not attack the worm at the core of the apple; it does not tackle the shadow side of fat issues, revealing the dark side of humanity, the side that seems to have a compulsion to victimise, to oppress, to stamp out. Big is Beautiful puts a forced smile on the face of fat without revealing the depths of unhappiness and humiliation that most fat women experience.[14]

Bovey criticises the creation of a dominant size rights culture of fashion and beauty which ignores the more painful aspects of being fat and traps fat people within photogenic but stereotyped 'super-achiever' roles, rather than dealing with fat oppression more realistically. Her attack also hints at the covert frictions between various size rights factions.

I think Bovey is a little harsh since many of us do find strength and affirmation from appearance, and it is fine for people to embrace frivolity, if that is what enables us to feel good and powerful. However, whilst 'Big is Beautiful' encompasses traditional areas of interest for women, such as beauty, and is therefore more accessible to many women than other kinds of politics or campaigning, like Bovey I am wary of a movement whose primary interest is based solely on appearances. This only reiterates the importance of how we look, not our abilities or personal qualities; it is shallow and conservative, about making ourselves acceptable, not changing the fundamental rules.

Bovey criticises 'Big is Beautiful' for being apologist, yet this is also a charge that has been directed at her. By the tone of her writing Bovey seems a good candidate for becoming a public fat rights figurehead. However, Bovey herself is ambivalent about her own fat body, and her behaviour appears in sharp contrast to the size acceptance ideas she promotes. In *The Forbidden Body*, Bovey describes rejoining Weight Watchers three years after *Being Fat is not a Sin* was first published. It is admirable that Bovey values honesty, I believe that her reservations about her body are representative of many fat people and, given the virulence of fat hatred, not surprising. However, I cannot pretend that I was not also saddened by her return to dieting.

For me, another disillusionment was Bovey's decision to change her book's title from *Being Fat is not a Sin* to *The Forbidden Body*.

This book was originally called *Being Fat is not a Sin*, a strong, factual statement, and it is still what this book is about. But many women are not ready to reclaim the word 'fat'. To stand in a bookshop in front of a strange sales assistant and ask for that title was too much for some. It meant drawing attention to their size and naming it, and using the F-word in the process! What was worse was that I, the author, was beginning to find that the title stuck in my throat whenever I was asked what my book was called. Fat activists will not approve of my evasive behaviour and I apologise to them, but being fat is so painful, such a sensitive issue for so many that I believe we must keep that in mind at all times.[15]

Bovey is sensitively tuned to those fat women amongst us who are beginning a struggle to find self-acceptance, and whom she seeks to protect. This is commendable, but I regard the name change as a retrograde step, like jumping back into the closet. With the title change, Bovey has disowned those of us who can and do use 'fat' to describe ourselves and to inform our politics – are we so atypical? I remember the first private thrill of pride and defiance I felt when I knew people could see me reading *Being Fat is not a Sin* in public, which others will not now enjoy. I empathise with Bovey's discomfort in discussing her book under its previous title – sometimes it feels very risky for me to mention my interest in fat politics with strangers and new friends – but I also feel that it is wrong to deny such a central aspect of my life. Although being out and open exposes me to potential ridicule, it also enables me to find allies in unexpected places. I do not want to live my life in fear, so instead of adopting a camouflage, I feel that it is more fruitful to develop assertive ways of protecting myself.

Shelley Bovey suffered hostile and insensitive media attention when *Being Fat is not a Sin* was first published, although her torment opened a new market for similar books. Margaret Greaves and Sue Dyson cover much the same ground as Bovey in their books, *Big and Beautiful* and *A Weight Off Your Mind*, although both have more of a self-help flavour. Bovey might criticise Greaves for being a representative of the Big is Beautiful Brigade, since there is a heavy reliance on fashion and beauty advice, complete with illustrations of curiously thin body types! Moreover, at the time of her publication Greaves was running 'Big and Beautiful' workshops. Her 'Fighting Back' recommendations, developed from these groups, is very individualistic; she urges fat women to dress well, develop a high self-esteem, and to lead a healthy lifestyle. Although Dyson refers to some aspects of the fat rights movement, Greaves does not acknowledge any collective efforts, such as NAAFA or the Fat Women's Group, as additional ways of challenging discrimination.

These divergent organisations in the US and in Britain represent the foundations upon which the present fat rights movement was built. Whilst the Fat Underground and *Extra Special* floundered, NAAFA and the Fat Women's Group have survived, albeit in changed forms that have had to take into account political differences and the rise in popularity of fat rights issues. All of these iniatives represent a courageous desire to break the silence and name fat hatred, even if that has meant speaking out in isolation and in the face of ridicule. Put simply, these groups and individuals took a big risk in order to make life better for other fat people.

Chapter Eight
The Fat Rights
Movement Today

Throughout *Fat and Proud* I have referred to a 'movement' of fat people and fat activists. The idea of a movement implies a group of people who come together, who have common aims and objectives, and who are mutually supportive. However, this is not a particularly accurate view of the fat rights movement. The recent secession of various local chapters from NAAFA has underscored long established divisions, and elsewhere many fat people are isolated, completely unaware that organisations promoting fat rights have existed for several decades. Fat rights issues have no one single organisational or theoretical foundation. Indeed, my fat rights activism developed because the traditional areas where I sought support, such as feminism or the politics of the left, were either failing to deal with fat issues adequately or ignoring them altogether. Because we have had to formulate our own frameworks for understanding fat hatred, we have relied heavily on pre-existing frameworks, such as the social model of disability, New Age spirituality, sexual politics, or medicine, and these are as diverse as our identities as fat people. Indeed, if cohesion is one's criterion for a movement, then perhaps the fat rights movement does not exist.

The idea of a unified size rights movement has only recently been created in order to compartmentalise the growth of interest in size rights issues, organisations, ideas and individuals. In reality there is no union and no global agenda, just many different factions. Fat activists and fat people comprise a community that is geographically, socially and politically diverse, and in many cases individuals, organisations and networks do not overlap with each other. Our diversity creates an enormous mixture of aims and objectives, many of which are conflicting; for example, some individuals favour law reform for fat people, or assimilation, whilst others prefer direct action and a more radical grass roots activism. Constituents of the size rights movement are not always in agreement or support of one another, and such differences of opinion can lead to great divisions. Perhaps it is more realistic to consider the size rights movement as a collection of movements. Whilst it is true that most of us have roughly similar goals, for example, an end to discrimination against fat people, we also have different ways of achieving those ends.

Below is a description of some of the organisations which comprise the movement, and some of the issues they address. Unless otherwise noted, most of these initiatives are North American, and towards the end of the chapter I discuss some of the cultural differences which influence fat activism in Britain and Stateside.

Professionals

Fat activism features the work of various people with a professional interest in fat issues. These people include health workers and administrators, sociologists, psychologists and other mental health professionals. Some professionals are active as writers, and others through the organisations in which they participate. Their research papers, articles, forums and debates help raise public consciousness around fat rights issues and help bring about the conditions necessary for change.

Several Americans have made influential literary contributions to fat politics. Earlier I mentioned the papers written by psychologists Susan Wooley and Orland Wayne Wooley, which used material from and legitimised many of the ideas of the Fat Underground. In *Obesity and Women I – A Closer Look at the Facts*, the authors discuss contemporary medical treatments for 'obesity', they question the opinion that being fat is unhealthy, and criticise social attitudes concerning fat people, suggesting that medical treatment options that are currently available should be revised in favour of more empowering practices.[1] In *Obesity and Women II – A Neglected Feminist Topic*, Wooley and Wooley discuss fatness as an issue of interest to feminists. Using material by Aldebaran and the Fat Underground, they argue that being fat is an ethical or political concern, as opposed to a medical, psychiatric or behavioural problem. In another ground-breaking paper, *Rethinking Obesity*, medical doctors Ernsberger and Haskew criticise conventional medical wisdom about fat people, and they contribute a non-judgemental and detailed outline of the health risks and benefits of being fat.[2] Today, Ernsberger uses much of the information gathered for *Rethinking Obesity* to train student doctors about size issues. Sociologist Hillel Schwartz has written a history of dieting in the US, linking current weight-loss fads and attitudes towards fatness with the fasts of religious aesthetes, and the growth of capitalism.[3] Laura Brown and Esther D Rothblum include accounts of incorporating fat-positive attitudes into their work as psychotherapists in *Overcoming Fear of Fat*.[4]

Some resources are primarily focused towards professionals. One example of this is *The Healthy Weight Journal*, formerly known as *Obesity and Health*, published in America by Francie Berg of the Healthy Living Institute. The journal combines medical and sociological material which is aimed at health professionals working amongst fat people. Contributors are basically critical of dieting and yo-yo weight gain, although some have yet to question their negative attitudes towards fat people, or relinquish their beliefs in the benefits of weight loss.

There have also been several organisations set up by lay activists to lobby professionals and seek their support. The Association For the Health Enrichment of Large People (AHELP) was founded by Dr Joe McVoy to educate professionals about fat rights issues and to lobby for appropriate medical treatment and research into fat people's health. The Council On Size and Weight Discrimination attempts to influence public policy and opinion in order to end fat oppression, and the Size Acceptance Network (SAN), based in South Australia, was established in 1993 to improve resources and opportunities for self-empowerment for people at all stages of 'the dieting-eating-disorder continuum'.

The involvement of professionals as organisers and activists is useful to the fat rights movement because the public views their perspective as being objective and therefore they legitimise the 'subjective' demands made by fat people. However, as I have pointed out in earlier chapters, there is an ambivalence for fat people in the power of professionals, especially medical professionals. Do grass roots ideas necessarily have to be filtered through a layer of professionals in order to make them legitimate and acceptable, especially if that group has a history of undermining and disempowering us as fat people? It is reassuring to have the backing of some professionals, but I would suggest that the movement should retain its diverse approach, relying on a multiplicity of voices whilst maintaining connections to fat people on the front line.

Campaigners

The aims of initiatives which feature the work of professionals can be allied to those of another group of fat rights activists: campaigners. Both groups seek to influence public opinion in favour of fat people, and bring to light issues which have an impact on our lives. They actively support changes in legislation and participate in public debates – representatives from the Council on Size and Weight Discrimination, for example, sat in on the pre-release hearings for dexfenfluramine (see p 106) to ensure that a fat rights perspective was given when decisions were made about the drug. Campaigners may act as individuals at grass roots level or form organisations such as Largesse, the Body Image Task Force, *Rump Parliament* and SIZE.

Largesse is based in Connecticut. Its directors, Karen W and Richard Stimson have become archivists and historians of the fat rights movement, particularly of feminist initiatives. Although it does not have close physical contact with its members through regular meetings, Largesse covers a huge geographical area and connects people through different channels of communication, such as by telephone, letter, e-mail or the World Wide Web. Largesse acts as a focal point for activists around the world to access information about fat issues, which enables people to direct their own campaigns. This service also helps support networks which already exist find each other and expand.

The Body Image Task Force was established by Dawn Atkins, a member of NAAFA's Research Committee. In

1988 Atkins was then also a member of the Santa Cruz Chapter of the National Organisation for Women (NOW), whom she challenged to officially oppose discrimination against fat people. NOW is a large and powerful organisation, and their recognition of fat issues was an important step for fat women. The California Chapter voted in favour of the change, but the Task Force split from NOW before the amendment finally entered its constitution.

Established in 1991, *Rump Parliament* is the work of Lee Martindale, who is based in Texas. *Rump Parliament* is a small press magazine which features news and information assembled to encourage groups and individuals to take action. For example, outside the state of Michigan fat people are not protected by anti-discrimination legislation in the workplace, and in 1997 Martindale launched Project Legislation 2000 in an attempt to add the category of weight to such statutes in the US. Much of the news in *Rump Parliament* is science-based, reflecting the medical attention given to fat people. As the US Coordinator of International No Diet Day, Martindale actively encourages people to hold public events to gain publicity for size issues. *Rump Parliament* also awards the annual Rumpie Awards to organisations and individuals who have influenced size rights, both positively and negatively.

So far campaigning organisations have been based in the US. However, SIZE, the National Size Acceptance Coalition, was established in Britain in 1996 by Diana Pollard and Tracey Jannaway of the Fat Women's Group. A networking coalition, it is still new at the time of writing and has yet to prove itself.

Groups which seek to influence attitudes towards fat issues are often run by charismatic and articulate individuals. These people voluntarily take on huge work-loads and responsibility, with, in most cases, little financial reward. Some campaigning organisations are rather capricious. An *ad hoc* gathering of fat activists on the East Coast of America known as the Fat Guerrillas carried out Operation Bookmark in 1995. They infiltrated bookshops and placed fat-acceptance and non-diet information between the pages of diet books on sale. Campaigners succeed in publicising important issues, and often they are responsible for determining what the focus of the movement should be. These groups are self-supporting. Their independence and self-sufficiency from fat community giants such as NAAFA is valuable because it enables them to be critical without fear of dismissal. The energy of campaigning groups is attractive, as is their broad-based inclusion of issues often eclipsed by more mainstream debates.

Support Groups

Trying to reverse the terrible psychological effect of living in fat-hating cultures by ourselves can be overwhelming, and many fat people need the support of others going through similar experiences, or the inspiration of those who have found peace and self-acceptance. Support prevents us from feeling isolated, and can be vital for fat people with eating disorders, fat people dealing with harassment or those recovering from a lifetime of dieting. Support groups also provide a way of sharing information and educating ourselves about fat rights issues.

There are different styles and types of support group. Some are very formal, others less so, and some organise using leaders, whilst others do not. Present-day support groups for fat people have their roots in the discussion and problem-solving style of the Fat Underground, which in turn was influenced by early feminist consciousness-raising groups. Such groups offer self-help resources for fat people to increase self-esteem, sometimes using group therapy techniques, with or without facilitators. These groups help participants to come to terms with being fat, and to get off the dieting treadmill.

The purpose of support groups is wide and varied. Some

offer services such as clothes-swapping networks; others organise demonstrations, workshops and newsletters. The groups also fulfil a social function where members can make new contacts. Groups may be self-financed or affiliated to larger organisations. In addition to these chapters there is a new strain of support group which has formed as a result of groups seceding from NAAFA. Many fat rights initiatives are located on the American coasts, and in capital cities. NAAFA has regional chapters, but there are also some independent regional support groups. Regional groups serve the needs of fat people who might otherwise be isolated from activities based on the coasts, and they also exist to create a local fat-positive community. Many support groups produce their own newsletters so that people living outside their geographical areas can subscribe and keep abreast of local news and issues. A basic tenet of support groups is that they create a safe space where individuals can be free to explore various issues. Many support groups have a feminist tradition, are informed by identity politics, and try to be accessible to particular social groups, such as lesbian women or people of colour, who are often marginalised and made invisible in mainstream organisations.

Support groups use small pockets of resources to fight for big ideas. Some groups are more successful than others at sustaining their activities and sense of direction to achieve their goals, and avoiding burn-out. Like all groups of people who come together to deal with a particular issue, there is often conflict amongst group members, or else different groups represent competing interests, and as a result some groups fizzle out, others appear, whilst some are long-standing. The diversity represented by support groups is a vibrant aspect of the grass roots struggle for fat rights, and support groups offer the potential to address everybody's needs, as well as the opportunity for different groups to build coalitions and develop an understanding of each other.

The Non-Diet Movement

Two realisations about dieting have created another movement that is strongly allied with fat rights activism. First, although not everybody is fat, most women in Anglo-American culture have experienced dieting, or have wanted to lose weight. Secondly, professionals and lay people have noticed that weight-loss diets are not effective, that they jeopardise one's health. Yo-yo dieting has been recognised as a major cause of ill-health, and there is a greater understanding of eating disorders.

Some people regard size acceptance as part of the non-dieting movement. They argue that individuals learn size acceptance and develop increased self-esteem as a result of stopping dieting and learning healthier ways of living. Others consider a non-dieting approach as a sub-group within the fat rights movement – fat politics encompasses many different aspects of our lives, and stopping dieting is only a part of fat people's struggles with fatphobia. The politics of dieting appeals to a broader audience of people than just those who are fat, so fat rights and non-diet initiatives have joined together. As well as these connections anti-diet groups also have links with consumer organisations, trading standards officials, food campaigners and researchers. Some governments have taken notice of dieting issues, for instance Canada and Norway have health promotion programmes which incorporate non-diet arguments.

Dietitians and psychotherapists are at the forefront of the non-dieting movement in the US and Canada. Many of them have lost faith in traditional approaches to fat people and dieting, and instead have tried to integrate 'diet recovery' and size-acceptance practices into their work. Some professionals have devised their own non-diet programmes, including workshops which are marketed as an alternative to diet clubs, such as Abundia and You*Nique.

Non-diet activism in Britain is channelled through Mary

Evans Young and Dietbreakers. Evans Young started Dietbreakers in 1991, inspired by her personal experience as a recovered dieter, and her professional life as a political campaigner and management consultant. Evans Young's biggest achievement has been the creation of International No Diet Day, an annual day in which people call a halt to dieting and weight obsession and bring public awareness to non-diet and size rights issues. It is also a celebratory day where alternatives to dieting are vigorously promoted. Evans Young first convened No Diet Day on 5 May 1992 as a picnic-cum-press-conference at her London home, featuring a group of supportive friends and relatives. By 1993 'International' had been added as a prefix because of the support Evans Young had received for her idea from the US. During this year she introduced the blue ribbon International No Diet Day symbol, having been inspired by the popularity and effect of the red AIDS awareness ribbons. In 1994 the event had grown into a rally with performers and speeches, but a year later the 1995 International No Diet Day Extravaganza planned in conjunction with *Yes!* magazine was cancelled because of high ticket prices and low sales. However, in the meantime International No Diet Day has taken off in the US, where long-established networks and fat rights activists have created a mass of events and coalitions to mark the day. International No Diet Day (now 6 May) is reaching people in more countries thanks to these efforts.

Evans Young has still maintained a high media profile for herself, Dietbreakers and non-diet issues through interviews, articles and a BBC Open Space documentary. In 1993 she began the first of her engagements with Alice Mahon, MP for Halifax, in an attempt to introduce British anti-diet legislation. Mahon became the mouthpiece for Dietbreakers, presenting an Early Day Motion (EDM) to the House of Commons in support of International No Diet Day. Despite the support of 73 MPs for the EDM, in 1994 Mahon's Ten Minute Rule Bill to regulate the diet industry failed. However, more recently both she and Evans Young have tried again to introduce legislation, this time to standardise dress sizes. Evans Young is also a business-woman and owner of the British franchise to a commercial non-diet course, The HUGS Programme, initiated in Canada. In addition she facilitates her own workshops, and has written a self-help book, *Dietbreaking*.

Some non-diet proponents are fatphobic, and do not support the fat rights movement. Whilst criticising the effects of dieting they are still in favour of weight loss as a healthy option, especially for fat people.[5] They operate a double standard, believing that dieting is only inap-propriate for thinner people, or sometimes those who are only a few pounds 'overweight'. Consequently, non-diet initiatives are having a curious effect on dieting and weight-loss advocates. Groups have changed the names of their diets to 'healthy eating plans', without disturbing any of the contents, or questioning their aspirations. Other businesses have appeared, such as the Weight Control Without Dieting workshops run in Britain by Genevieve Blais who criticises dieting but has no qualms about weight-control programmes.

Other initiatives are size-positive. Some non-diet workshop providers include and acknowledge fat people, they work in coalitions with fat activists, especially around events such as International No Diet Day, and many non-diet professionals use their status to support fat rights. For example, some women working in and around Harlow in Essex include non-diet and size rights issues as part of their professional repertoire in counselling projects at the local Well Women Centre and in programmes involving young people. In the early 1990s Heavenly Bodies was a support group in Harlow attended by some fat women which attempted to help women question attitudes to food, their bodies, dieting, the politics of beauty, and healthy living. Heavenly Bodies no longer exists but it was the catalyst for other local non-diet initiatives, such as the Women, Food and Feelings Working Group who have organised workshops and community conferences addressing dieting and size acceptance.

Products and Services

Recently a consumer revolution has been named by the British media. Apparently people are demanding products and services which more accurately reflect their needs and interests. Manufacturers and retailers are discovering that they are having to be more accountable to their consumers. As fat people become less apologetic about our size, we are also beginning to demand products and services which suit us, rather than forcing ourselves to use items which do not fit us or are unsuitable.

Clothes

North American shops offer a wider range of sizes and cater to more varied clothing markets than their counterparts in Britain. Here, most large towns have at least one high street chain shop or department store which sells large sizes. Many of these have restyled their large-size departments, moving away from old 'Outsize' connotations, which women found embarrassing and exclusive, to introduce more fashionable lines. But despite a wealth of places to buy larger-sized clothes compared to ten years ago, retailers in both America and Britain are reluctant to include super-sizes, and larger fat women still have a problem buying clothes to fit. Elsewhere, some companies are beginning to feature celebrity endorsements by famous fat actresses – an unusual development, since such people are under a lot of showbusiness pressure to be thin. Smaller retailers are generally more in touch with their clientele. They tend to focus on quality and service, rather than cost and quantity, and often feature a greater spectrum of sizes. Some small retailers have been involved with the fat rights movement, speaking out in the media about size issues.

Products

There are now agencies which publicise and sell consumer goods specifically for a fat and super-sized market, such as large-sized sewing patterns, hammocks, wetsuits, seatbelt extenders, long coat-hangers and tape measures. Some businesses are a reaction to the discrimination fat people deal with in 'normal' surroundings. In Britain, for example, there are special dating agencies and nightclubs for fat people and Fat Admirers. Fat issues have also surfaced through independent publishing, whether blatantly activist, such as Diana Pollard's Rotunda Press, which produced a British edition of the American *Shadow on a Tightrope* anthology in the late 1980s, or more covertly so, such as the American Rubenesque Romances series which publishes traditional romantic fiction featuring fat heroines.

Until now consumer agencies and services for fat people have run along the lines of small cottage industries. At present, these small businesses are run by people who are dedicated to size rights, who have a personal stake in social change for fat people, and their involvement confers a sensitivity to their clients' needs. As the market expands, with fat people demanding more widespread and sophisticated services, larger businesses will want to buy a piece of the action. One wonders how they will respond to the needs and interests of their fat consumers, and what will happen to the smaller businesses. It is ironic that in creating a market for fat people, small fat activist-inspired companies may be putting themselves out of business.

Exercise

During the 1980s, fat activists on the West Coast of America pioneered sports and exercise activities that were accessible to fat people. Whilst the majority of fitness adherents were busily going for the burn in an attempt to streamline their bodies, a new wave of participants were using exercise in a different way. The work of Pat Lyons and Debby Burgard came to prominence through their articles in *Radiance: The Magazine for Large Women*, and their book *Great Shape*.[6] As fat women who were interested in sport and exercise, they organised exercise classes for others like them in California, combining their understanding of the social issues for fat women with ideas about fitness. Lyons and Burgard proposed that there was no reason fat people could not be fit; they suggested that health is an individually determined and subjective experience; and they stated that fat people should become knowledgeable about their own bodies instead of relying completely on distant experts and professionals. Lyons and Burgard suggested that exercise can be part of fat women's recovery from body hatred, eating disorders and dieting. As fat people it is important that we learn to enjoy exercise and movement now, not in some mythical future when we'll be thinner. Exercise can be playful and fun, it can be a pleasurable way of building self-confidence, learning body awareness and eliminating some of the shame we might feel towards ourselves.

Great Shape does not encourage us to rush out and buy a gym membership that we will never use. Instead, it suggests that we ease ourselves into movement slowly and find something to do that we enjoy, which could include a whole range of things from throwing away the television remote control, to weightlifting, or just walking. It suggests exercising alone, with friends, or as part of a larger group. Lyons and Burgard mention their involvement with We Dance which, like the swimming group Making Waves, was amongst the first exercise sessions that were specifically geared towards fat women. We Dance and Making Waves provided a space that was accessible, both in terms of financial cost and organisation. We Dance restricted its membership to women who weighed over 200lb (approximately 14 stone), whilst Making Waves sometimes held mixed sessions with thinner women. Members and organisers worked hard to make the classes non-judgemental and supportive by creating exercises that were suitable and safe for everyone. In

Britain this work has been carried on by community groups such as Fat and Fit in Newcastle-upon-Tyne.

As well as educating fat women about the effect of exercise on our fat bodies, We Dance, Making Waves and similar subsequent initiatives do not work on the premise that losing weight is the right reason for us to exercise. They have shown that this is another useful way for fat women to come together, have fun, and benefit from each other's company. Interestingly, this form is being purloined by slimming clubs. By its name alone, one would suspect the Large and Lovely Club, which meets at a sports centre in London, to be another fat-friendly exercise group. However, Large is not so Lovely at this group, which is for:

> Women who want to see changes in their physical appearance, yet feel too self-conscious to go to a class. Working holistically we will help you to understand why you find it difficult to lose weight, we will listen, support, and motivate you to make the changes you desire.[7]

Week three of the Large and Lovely Club introduces practical tips on reducing fat in one's diet, and all workshops include fat-burning and muscle-toning classes. I find it an interesting mark of how popular fat-positive exercise groups have become that their format is being appropriated by weight-loss proponents. It also highlights the conflict between the desire of fat rights advocates to create a place where fat people can take exercise without the pressure to lose weight and our own longing as fat people to be thinner.

Magazines
Women's magazines fulfil certain functions: whilst they can be criticised for reinforcing stereotyped behaviour, they also legitimise parts of our lives which are seen as trivial in other contexts, such as cooking and fashion; they

are a cheap and reliable treat; they offer support and advice to the reader, like a trusted friend; and they create a sense of community. Fat people are often relegated to the margins of society, and our experiences and the issues we deal with are also passed over as trivial. We need an accessible means of support so that we can create a positive identity for ourselves, and women's magazines are a good format by which to do this. Until the mid-80s the only magazines which featured fat people were those which promoted dieting. Since then, several attempts have been made to appropriate women's magazines, for example, *Radiance: The Magazine for Large Women*, an American title published by Alice Ansfield. In circulation since 1984, the first edition had a home-made appearance, similar to a zine (amateur publication), although today *Radiance* has evolved into a glossy bi-monthly. The magazine combines profiles of fat activists and professionals, media reports, a cooking column, resources, fashion, news, fiction and self-help advice about healthy living as fat people. In earlier years Ansfield organised Radiance Retreats which were events enabling fat women to come together and combine a holiday with fat-positive workshops and demonstrations. More recently Ansfield has revived this idea with Radiance Cruises to Alaska and the Caribbean.

Radiance sprang from a tradition of community newsletters and self-publishing, whereas size-acceptance magazines in Britain are influenced by the style of mainstream titles, and share more in common with US fashion magazines such as *Extra!* and *Big Beautiful Woman*. I have already mentioned *Extra Special*, and here are two more examples.

Pretty Big was published by Audrey Winkler between 1990 and 1995. It was an independent operation, sold by subscription, which graduated from a small black and white format to full-colour gloss. *Pretty Big* was almost entirely fashion orientated, directed towards individuals as well as people within the clothing industry, in which

Winkler is a vociferous lobbyist for larger sizes. Aside from the fashion, *Pretty Big* featured articles about fat role models and, being based in the Midlands, it reflected life for fat people away from the capital.

For most of its lifetime *Pretty Big* was a lone voice in the media for fat women, which is a big responsibility for a small press fashion magazine. Audrey Winkler's vision was not for everybody, and *Pretty Big* was criticised for not engaging in fat issues outside of fashion, and producing articles which were sketchy and a little tame. Ultimately the growth of *Yes!* heralded *Pretty Big*'s demise.

Janice Bhend launched *Yes!* in 1993. Bhend had previously written a large-size fashion column in *Woman's Weekly*, and was a regular contributor to *Extra Special*. *Yes!* is a glossy bi-monthly magazine, which reads like an updated *Extra Special*. It features regular women's magazine articles such as make-overs and advice, but has also lent its support to community events such as International No Diet Day. Many of the writers in *Yes!* are prominent size-acceptance advocates, and the magazine therefore reflects some of the current debates in the British movement.

Extra Special, *Pretty Big* and *Yes!* have raised the profile of fat issues and introduced them to new audiences. They translate fat politics into a form that is very accessible for many women. However, the tone and range of the material they can publish is affected by the interests of their advertisers, which ensure the magazines' economic survival. *Encore*, launched in 1996 and published on behalf of the clothes shop Evans Ltd, is little more than an extended infomercial. Therefore magazines may be unwilling to feature material, groups and individuals who do not fit the editorial policy, or the values that are promoted by the advertisers. Sometimes the worldview promoted by mainstream magazines can be a little bit too safe and cosy.

*

Arts and Entertainment

There have been always been fat women performers. Black jazz and blues singers have been named for their size, for example, Big Maybelle, Ma Rainey and Big Mama Thornton, and later the white pop singer Mama Cass Elliot. More recently The Weather Girls, previously known as Two Tons of Fun, have flaunted their bodies. Many fat performers make a joke of their fatness but lately, in the mainstream mass media and in smaller scale projects, fat people and fat rights issues are being addressed.

On television fat people are most often presented on talk shows or as comedians. Talk shows are directed at women and feature domestic subject matter such as relationships and resolving personal problems. Within this context these programmes frequently play host to fat people either as 'victims', experts, or slimmed down as diet evangelists or hosts (sometimes both). Many of us enjoy talk shows and find useful insights from them. However, despite the regular appearance of fat issues, and despite their popularity, these programmes are problematic. Fat people do not set the agenda; we appear only to fit into a predetermined and formulaic format featuring ourselves as sensationalised freaks. In talk shows nothing is ever really resolved, and complex problems are reduced to pithy and superficial soundbites. The producers and presenters present as sympathetic, but programmes about fat people are really about grabbing rating points.

Two comedians, Jo Brand and Dawn French have become very popular amongst some British fat activists, but others find their humour more problematic. At times it is difficult to establish whether the audience is laughing with them, or at them.

The appeal of large audiences for fat issues comes at the expense of having to work to an uneducated agenda, where many messages are toned down, where the same debates occur over and over again, or where double messages are issued about the acceptability of fat bodies. It is with

smaller scale projects that we can use arts and entertain-
ments to express our arguments more effectively, and they
sometimes catch the eye of a wider audience. Many fat
rights journals publish poetry and fiction, and now writers
such as Susan Stinson, the American author of *Fat Girl
Dances with Rocks* and *Martha Moody*, who bring a fat
activist sensibility to their work, are being courted by
mainstream retailers and book clubs.[8]

Theatre is a good example of how fat activist groups are
making use of the arts. Fat Lip Readers Theatre, based in
San Francisco, shares a historical connection to the
theatrical protests of the Fat Underground, and to groups
which stemmed from the Fat Underground, in particular
Fat Chance. Fat Chance was a dance and acrobatic troupe
founded by Leah Kushner and Judy Freespirit. The group
consisted of fat women who wanted a safe space in which
to dance and perform. Fat Chance split by the early 1980s,
but in 1982 Fat Lip Readers Theatre debuted with *For Fat
Women Only*. Readers' theatre is a type of performance
where actors read from scripts on-stage instead of
memorising lines. It is a good way of creating performance
pieces with people who have little performance
experience. The group meets and discusses what it wants
to do before formulating a play. Work is then written by
group members, or other contributors, often based on
personal experience, and integrated into the performance.
Fat Lip took inspiration from other readers' theatre groups
in the Bay Area in California, and included women who
were already actively involved in various fat rights
organisations alongside those who were just discovering
their interest. Fat Lip perform to restricted audiences of fat
women, as well as mixed-sized people, and in 1995 the
company toured with *Hot Lips: Sex and Chocolate*, a
performance piece about fat women and sexuality.

Activists are appropriating video technology to continue
the performance tradition. Fat Lip produced *Nothing to
Lose*, which used material from past performances. In
1989 the Boston Area Fat Liberation group made *Throwing*

Our Weight Around, in which group members discuss and act out everyday scenes highlighting some of the issues fat people deal with. More recently, in 1994, Canadian Rick Zakowich directed and starred in the full-length autobiographical documentary *Fat Chance: The Big Prejudice*. The video shows the progress of a fat man moving from dieting and self-hatred to self-acceptance and political activism. Also in 1994 I produced my own video, *Growing Up Fat 1983–1990*, which uses diary extracts and interviews to chart the formation of my identity as a young fat woman.

Photography is a popular medium amongst individual fat activist artists, most of whom produce images of fat bodies. During the 1980s Patricia Schwarz, an American independent fine art photographer, produced a series of images entitled *Women of Substance*, photographing fat women in settings traditionally associated with slender figures, such as in swimsuits and as classically posed nudes. Schwarz is an award winner, taking the 1986 French Agfa/Forum Dodation for her use of colour, and in 1989 she won the Ruttenberg Foundation Award with a photograph entitled *Fat Lady*.

More recently Laurie Toby Edison's photographs have appeared in the American book *Women En Large: Images of Fat Nudes*, alongside essays and prose by Debbie Notkin.[9] *Women En Large* has been praised for its depiction of a wide diversity of real fat women, its use of personal accounts by the models which accompany the images, and for the way the book pulls together political writing and photography.

Finally, in the visual arts in Britain, Rachael Field is a lesbian and an artist who paints images of herself as a fat woman. Her paintings are often very big. *Broadening Out* (1991) is a self-portrait with Field looking out of the canvas and waving her arms animatedly, whilst lower down a sequined button on her shirt has popped open. Field explains:

It's taking the piss out of myself but also hating it when

people laugh at me. It's putting that fat back into the cult image of the thin woman, trying to counter some of the body fascism and elitism in the lesbian culture, the lesbian scene. It's about demanding space, about taking space; allowing myself to get bigger within the work and saying, 'Hey, look at me! I'm lovely!'[10]

Zines

Zines are a great medium for fat activists, and several currently produced on both sides of the Atlantic focus on fat activism or other fat issues. A zine (rhymes with 'bean' not 'line') is:

A small handmade amateur publication done purely out of passion, rarely making a profit or breaking even.[11]

Zine culture in Britain and the States has grown out of the increased availability of relatively cheap publishing resources and new distribution networks. For example, *Living Large* is an amateur press association apa zine for fat people. An apa is an interactive zine, created by a group of subscribers. Participants submit work which is gathered together by a central mail collector, photocopied and published. Since *Living Large* participants live all over the US, and since I contribute from Britain, the effect is of reading an international meeting between up to twenty different fat people.

Zines differ from mainstream magazines because they are usually created by individuals instead of companies, and zine creators do not always employ high production values or profit margins, which makes them cheap. Zines have low print runs and even the most popular have small distribution numbers compared to newspapers and magazines. Unlike the mainstream press only the larger zines carry advertising, and this is usually restricted to individuals and businesses within the zine's own community. This policy enables zine producers to exercise a freedom of opinion that is unfettered, unlike mainstream magazines, which must protect their advertisers' interests in order to benefit from advertising revenue. For example, *i'm so fucking beautiful* is produced by Nomy Lamm, who is young, fat, disabled, lesbian and Jewish, and the zine is greatly influenced by riot grrl, a North American movement of young women reclaiming feminism with a do-it-yourself/punk ethos. Lamm uses *i'm so fucking beautiful* as an outlet to explore and educate people about personal issues such as growing up fat and coming to terms with her body, although in recent editions she addresses the political context of fat oppression. Lamm is frequently angry, raw and uncompromising, in i*'m so fucking beautiful 2¹/₂* she rants:

> This zine is for those of you with skinny privilege. and this is the LAST time that I'm gonna point out yr privilege/fucking abusiveness for you. (yeah right nomy) yeah again and again i've found that i'm the only one i know the only one around who's gonna always be dealing with FAT OPPRESSION. YEAH everyone knows that when there's something sizeist, nomy's the one to tell. nomy's the one who will do something about it. ask nomy what to do. or just sit around and wait to see what nomy will do. I AM NOT A WALL OF STEEL. I DON'T ALWAYS KNOW WHAT TO DO (I DON'T ever know what to do . . .) i know that you are working on your sizeism, i know that you support me and understand me. but does it only go as far as your interactions with me? i don't know what i'm saying. i don't know anything.

Lamm's honesty and provocativeness makes a startling change from the calm and professional tone of many fat rights organisations.

Because of their independence and accessibility, zines express an eclectic range of subject matter, often representing the values of marginalised communities, for example, sex and political radicals, who are not covered in the mainstream press. *Fat!So?*, a San Francisco zine edited by Marilyn Wann uses streetwise humour to address fat politics, throwing in knowing references to fat rights iconography by publishing, for example, a Venus of Willendorf paper cut-out dress-up doll, a flicker book showing Oprah's weight yo-yo-ing wildly, or subverting the standard diet pledge which begins so many weight-loss regimes:

> Fat!So? invites YOU to be a fabulous fatso! Everybody: Size 6 to 16. Size 26 to 56. Because fat or thin, straight or gay, male or female, we have all at some point wasted our precious moments on the planet worrying about how we look. Fuck that! Just say the magic words: 'Yes, I am a fatso!' Write it here in the space provided:
> ....With these words you create revolution. You turn fat hatred back on itself. As a fatso, you possess the ultimate weapon against fatphobia, body prejudice, and size oppression: fatso pride![12]

Unlike their American counterparts, the British zines that have included material about fat politics address fat issues alongside other concerns, they are not primarily fat activist. For example, in 1993 *GirlFrenzy* published a special fat politics issue with articles and comic strips. Other zines such as *Red Hanky Panky* and *Lone Star Comics* have an active interest in fat issues and feature fat characters, and Lee Kennedy's comics frequently discuss her personal struggles with weight loss and fat hatred.

On-line Activism

The development of the internet has facilitated the spread of ideas both between activist groups and individuals. One of the main advantages of the net is the freedom of expression and freedom of information which, considering the cultural mythology that surrounds fat people, is very useful. The internet gives us access to a mass of information and perspectives that are critical and challenging of fat hatred through newsgroups and discussion forums such as alt.support.big-folks.

Being on-line is a means of overcoming geographical distance instantaneously and very cheaply, which means that it is a useful means of communication for fat people who are physically isolated, for example, through impaired mobility or a lack of local resources. Moreover, new virtual communities are being established, for example, through specialised e-mail lists such as *Fatdykes*, an international group of, surprise, fat dykes! Here individuals can find support, locate information and take part in debates relevant to the particular group. One concern here is that when shared identity becomes the sole focus of a community, groups split off into smaller and smaller factions, sometimes competing with each other. This begs questions such as what happens to the wider struggle – is it abandoned, or does it take a new form in these smaller groups? Are our identities an endless quarry? What is there to say to each other after the quest for identity has been exhausted? Have we split off because of our fear of negotiating difference? Meanwhile, the nature of the net is a challenge to notions of exclusivity: some e-mail lists struggle to filter out people they don't want, for example, it is very easy to camouflage one's gender on-line and therefore very difficult to exclude men from women-only spaces.

The World Wide Web can be a useful resource since many fat rights activists, publications and groups have their own websites detailing their activities. Fat-related FAQs, sites listing Frequently Asked Questions and responses around a given subject, are also accessible. These sites tend to be regularly updated with fresh information and are good places to find out about basic fat rights issues. There is a 'no experts' principle implicit, and information posted there by web users, and also in news and e-mail groups, is usually based on personal experience, practical and down-to-earth in tone. On the other hand the web is becoming increasingly commercialised, sites have become complex advertisements and infomercials designed to shift products, rather than being altruistic resources.

Freedom of expression on the net and its unregulated nature also mean that information is difficult to verify, or it becomes undermined by gossip and hearsay. Many users complain about having to sift through drifts of babble or irrelevant material before they find anything useful. For the time being, of course, the hardware needed to access the internet is expensive, a luxury item beyond the means of most people, and the medium remains the domain of an exclusive few.

America v. Britain

Why are so many of these initiatives based in North America? Generally speaking, much of the American material I read seems very radical in comparison to that from Britain. Here we do not have the same number of organisations as do American fat activists, neither are we as professionally organised in general as many of their groups, so there is a tendency for us to regard ourselves as poor backward cousins in comparison. In Europe several national groups for fat people exist but our different languages make it difficult for us to network with one another. However, whilst Britain and America share a similar language, we are very different cultures, and the activism in our respective countries is influenced by these differences.

The size rights movement in Britain is much younger than in the US. There is no national association comparable to NAAFA, so we work without the support of a large and powerful organisation. British groups are almost wholly voluntary, with little prospect of long-term funding. The smallness and solitude of fat activism in Britain means that many individuals promote only their own agendas, and the same pundits pop up time and time again rather than representatives of a more varied movement. However, fat activists in Britain are also pioneers, our relative inexperience allows us a sense of freedom to find our own voices, rather than conforming to somebody else's system. Neither are we completely alone and without support; we are in an enviable position of being free to form our own movement whilst being able to learn from the examples set by American organisations.

Diet industries in Britain are a shadow of those in the States. We do not have diet centres in almost every shopping mall. America churns out a new diet guru every year, from Jack LaLanne, to Richard Simmons, to Susan Powter, but thankfully in Britain we only really have to suffer the perennial Rosemary Conley. Like pro-choice and anti-abortion politics, fat activists and diet proponents are polarised in the US. As fat rights has become more recognisable and influential, and fat people have won legal fights against diet companies and products which have ruined their health, diet industries have become threatened and protect their businesses more aggressively. In Britain there is less of a deadlock, perhaps because the debates are less familiar to us. Because the boundaries of fat people involved with fat politics as well as dieting and weight loss practices are very fluid, there is more of a dialogue between the different groups. Often this results in muddle, but it also enables British fat activists to reach an audience that is cut off to our American counterparts.

Chapter Nine
All Together Now?

The fat rights movement has many goals, from legal advances to personal empowerment for all fat people. Fat rights advocates want to experience a positive change in attitude towards fat people, we want respect, and most of us want to destroy the assumption that fat people should be, and want to be, thin. However, these are value-laden desires; what is positive for one person may not be for another, respect can mean many things, and we have already found that a majority of fat people, even amongst activists, still desire weight loss. It seems we may all be struggling for very different goals under a veneer of shared beliefs.

That there is no singular and unified movement is regarded as a problem by some people because it suggests in-fighting and destructive competition; it implies that our goals are indistinct and therefore untenable; and irreconcilable differences threaten any coalitions we might make. Many fat activists seem keen to promote the notion of a global size rights movement because not to do so implies that we are politically ineffectual. Some of us worry about how we might be construed by outsiders, we are a relatively new and therefore inexperienced movement and we do not want to advertise our vulnerability – would it be used to discredit us? In the mainstream little is known about us and when we do get coverage we are represented as cranks or as a freakshow. Sometimes fat activists try and present all members of the size rights movement as people who have totally and successfully come to terms with being fat; it is easier to sell the benefits of fat rights activism to a sceptical public if we overlook the complexities and contradictions with which fat people really deal.

However, the fact that we are not a unified movement does not diminish our power. Our diversity presents a sophisticated response to the perniciousness of fat hatred, and the variety within fat rights initiatives and ideas ensures that there is a place for everyone. Fat people bring many values to our activism and this should be a source of pride; maintaining a broad front enables fat people to fight and exert influence over a wide variety of areas. There is nothing distasteful about the truth – that we do not always have much in common with each other beyond our body sizes – but our differences need to be addressed and not swept under the carpet. This will enable fat people to develop a more realistic awareness of fat rights issues rather than shuttering out what we think does not apply to us. This is the groundwork that will help build coalitions, and help us work together with mutual respect without compromising individual identities and values.

Sources of Conflict

The mythology of a cohesive fat rights movement, and the fear of differences or complexities within it has led to the promotion of some beliefs which threaten to undermine its integrity. What follows are some examples. First, an assumed homogeneity has created grossly over-simplified and distorted analyses of historical and cross-cultural perspectives regarding fatness, where important details have been airbrushed away for the sake of a snappy soundbite. Secondly, prejudice within the movement endangers the tenets of size rights.

Historical perspectives

Many fat activists cite historical and cross-cultural differences between attitudes to fatness because they are evidence that fat hatred in twentieth-century Anglo-American cultures is not inevitable. However, these analyses are often very clumsy.

Often we take from history only what we want to see, only material which fits our modern size rights perspective. Many fat people, for example, refer to the historical period which is represented in the paintings of Peter Paul Rubens (1577–1640) as a utopia, where fat women were valued and adored. It is comforting to find evidence documenting a time where we imagine that fat women were revered instead of despised. However, when we do this we are avoiding important details. Rubens painted women not as autonomous beings but as symbols representing moral concepts such as virtue. This is an artistic discourse which is not concerned with representing everyday normality. Therefore his images cannot be cited as solid proof that fat women had higher status then compared to now. Rubens painted during a time when women were hardly emancipated, indeed, I regard his renditions of us as very passive and powerless, not exactly empowering role models for women today. The fat women in Rubens' paintings, and other works of that period are not very fat; their bodies follow a particular pattern of small breasts, round pot bellies, and fleshy hips, but they do not represent a wide range of fat body types. Rubens was an artisan for the upper classes and his representations of beauty embodied in fat women reflected the values of the ruling class, on which his livelihood depended. The ruling classes have always been estranged from the majority of the population, and their values are not always representative of the times. Hence I believe that the images of fat women in these paintings are exclusive and perpetuate the belief that there can only ever be one standard of beauty for women's bodies, which in this case happens to be a bit fat, instead of liberating everybody from such restrictions.

We tend to refer to historical evidence with twentieth-century values. The Venus of Willendorf is a good example of this process. The Venus of Willendorf is a prehistoric statue of a symbolic fat woman. Fat activists have described her as a goddess, a depiction of prehistoric beauty and fecundity. However, we cannot confirm these labels, neither can we know the real significance of the Venus of Willendorf, and other similar artifacts, for the historical communities which produced them. Given fat activists' record of simplifying other historical periods, I am sceptical that our readings of the Venus of Willendorf are much more than projections of our desire to find ourselves in the past.

Other historical analyses continue through more recent accounts involving discussions about filmstars and models and whether they represent periods of comparative fat liberation or oppression. Particular favourites for debate are the 'mammary goddesses' of the American 1950s, such as Marilyn Monroe, who is said to have been a size 16, supposedly proving the argument that in the past one could be fat and considered a great beauty (yet she also dieted regularly and her body size varied dramatically); Twiggy, who by many accounts is responsible for an epidemic of anorexia; and latterly the supermodel phenomenon.

The historical evidence cited by fat people in order to support size rights theories tends to be condensed into over-simplified periods which reduce rich and complex issues into sanitised, culturally indistinct, easily referenced compartments. This is little more than a romanticised and simplified view of the past based on a very small number of touchstone images and selective representations. We filter out any material which does not fit our theories about fat people then and now. I am not attempting to debunk all our beliefs about historical differences between people's attitudes to fatness, but if we want to use historical arguments intelligently and convincingly I suggest that we begin to consider some important details. This entails asking questions about the context of historical references, for example, whose perspective they represent and how relevant is this to us now? We should consider what we are trying to illustrate by reading a figure or an era in one particular way, as well as reconciling rather than ignoring material which does not fit with our ideology. In doing this, I doubt we will find cartoonish icons, or uncover evidence as dramatic as we would like, more likely we will find similar cultural ambivalence towards fatness as we experience now. I do believe, however, that an increased sensitivity will result in material that more accurately reflects a realistic picture of what fat represents.

Cross-cultural analyses

Attitudes vary cross-culturally and this, not surprisingly, includes attitudes towards fatness which are not as infused with fear and hatred as they are in Anglo-American societies. This is a difficult theory to prove. There are arguments put forward to suggest it is true, but these are both questionable and complicated. The belief that some cultures admire and appreciate fatness makes fat people in Britain and America feel more comfortable, it is used to support fat rights arguments that fatness is not necessarily ugly, whatever the reality is for people living within the cultures described.

The basic premise is that in some cultures, usually in Africa or the Caribbean, fatness is desirable in women since it connotes abundance where food is scarce. A fat woman becomes a kind of trophy who symbolises a family's wealth and status in its success in being able to feed itself. I am not presenting evidence here to demonstrate that in some non-Anglo-American cultures fat is valued and accepted because I do not have that proof. Instead I wish to discuss the arguments which suggest it is true; arguments which are questionable and complicated.

Cultural differences have not been documented extensively or convincingly by writers, researchers and activists investigating fat issues, and the use of cross-cultural arguments to show that fatphobia is not inevitable is problematic. In my research I have found that much of this evidence is based on hearsay and isolated individual experiences, whilst longer accounts of fat people in 'other cultures' are often supplied by Anglo-American women travelling as tourists, aid workers and anthropologists, such as Margaret Mead in Western Samoa, rather than by fat women from the cultures in question. I wonder how much evidence is being distorted or read out of context in order to fit size rights theories.

Sometimes the belief that being fat is acceptable in 'other cultures' assumes that many diverse cultures are homogenous, or fit a black/white binary opposition, that there might not also be differences of attitudes in cultures within cultures, and this encourages Anglo-American fat activists to make vast generalisations. Sue Dyson, for example, does this with statistics, pointing out that 81 per cent of the world's cultures 'still believe that overall plumpness or moderate fatness is desirable in women', and that 90 per cent find fat hips and thighs attractive'.[1] She does not source this reference, it alludes only to 'moderate' fatness rather than fat people of all sizes, and she does not define what she means by 'world's cultures' – are they delineated by race, or country, or socio-economic group, or some other boundary? How valid is the methodology used to gather this information?

As with historical analyses, beliefs about fat people in modern cultures other than those that are white-majority are similarly insensitive and sexist, where women are again dehumanised as symbols with no voice of their own, and where to be considered beautiful by men is regarded as the ultimate goal. Few of the cultures that are usually mentioned as having a more accepting attitude to fat women, such as in Africa or the Caribbean, have massive and permanent problems with famine or drought; a belief that they do is myth, so how does this affect the assumption that fat people are symbols of plentitude? That fat people supposedly embody an abundance of food is questionable, especially since many fat activists have been insisting from the very beginning that fat people eat no more than those who are thinner. If fat people are thought to represent a large appetite for food, where does that leave debates in favour of a genetic explanation of fatness, and of set point theory? The notion of women as trophies or possessions is deplorable, especially when this is based on our appearance or body size. Fat or thin, should fat rights advocates really be celebrating cultures where one body type is honoured at the expense of another? It may be, of course, that developing cultures are more sophisticated and do not depend on the either/or philosophy which permeates Anglo-American society; perhaps such cultures celebrate beauty and desirability across the board. Beliefs about fat people in other cultures focus exclusively on fat women; if a whole culture is under scrutiny, why are the men absent, and what does this mean? Lastly, it is false to think of cultures which have a different attitude to fat women than the one we are used to as utopian. Some cultures in West Africa, such as in Mauritania and

Northern Mali, practise force-feeding of girls and women as a rite of passage which accompanies such life events as female genital mutilation, marriage or motherhood. Women's organisations have criticised this practice as degrading and health-threatening, although since many people regard it as a traditional custom, force-feeding has been difficult to challenge.[2] Hardly a Garden of Eden!

Fat activists in white-majority cultures may take comfort from the knowledge that fatness is not regarded in the same way everywhere. However, fat people of colour and non-Western or Anglo-American societies are nevertheless compartmentalised as different and somehow separate from the rest of 'us'. It is as though the myth that 'they' have a positive view of fat women is such a strong source of affirmation that we do not want it shattered, we do not want to examine the reality. This encourages white size rights activists to ignore the reality for people of colour, and to avoid considering the campaign for fat rights as a movement with global implications.

The fat rights movement is dominated by white people, few of whom are considering ethnicity in their work. White cultural ethnocentrism is for me one of the major drawbacks of the fat rights movement. It angers me that we claim a tradition alongside other civil rights movements yet we fail to recognise the needs and demands of the originators of those movements. Aside from the most superficial comments about fatness being acceptable in 'other' cultures, there has been no real mention of what fatness means to different communities. Debates about the significance of fatness and ethnicity are sorely needed, which not only concern descendants of Africa, but also include other people of colour such as Asians, Arabs, Latin and Native Americans, and particularly people from cultures which appear to have a more positive acceptance of fatness such as Pacific Island communities.

Prejudice
Incongruously, for a movement which seeks to free people

from prejudice based on one's appearance, new standards of 'looksism' are being established, and these ideals feature a distinct fear of bodily difference.

Fat people's definitions of 'fat' make a big impact on debates about who should be included in, and excluded from, the size rights movement. Although the issues addressed by the fat rights movement concern most people regardless of size, this is an autonomous movement generated by fat people to serve our interests. As I pointed out in the introduction, there are problems with the various definitions of who is fat, so there are no concrete rules governing who can be a member. This makes some fat activists uncomfortable. There is some ambivalence towards smaller fat people within the movement, who are regarded as less oppressed and therefore less able to assert a claim on fat liberation. There is also animosity towards thinner people in general, women in particular, and 'skinny', 'stick insect', and 'anorexic' have become terms of abuse. This is often combined with ignorance about eating disorders and fostered by a desire to distance fat people from being labelled, as we often are, in terms of dysfunctional eating habits. Moreover, some fat people express anger that sufferers of anorexia 'get all the attention' in terms of service provision and sympathy, as opposed to fat people, who are blamed and vilified for our fatness. Yet, as I have said, fatness is a body size, anorexia is a dysfunctional coping strategy, therefore it is right that sufferers of eating disorders should have access to help and healthcare. The hatred of thinner people is fostered by fat people's anger at fat oppression and the drawing of battle lines opposite those who are assumed to be complicit with fat oppression. But thinner people are a false target; people can be fatphobic at any size, being fat exempts nobody. Not all thinner people hate and fear us, and our animosity is alienating; we are perpetuating thinner people's ignorance of our lives, losing potential allies, and denying acceptance of body diversity.

It is not only thinner people who are under attack.

Within groups of fat people new divisions are forming. The well-worn statistic which asserts that 47 per cent of British women wear a size 16 or larger is often quoted by size rights proponents because it implies that there is a huge and potentially powerful population of fat people in Britain. Although nearly half of British women wear a size 16 or larger, as dress size increases, the percentage of women rapidly diminishes. Therefore although there are a great many women who wear a dress size larger than the standard 10/12/14 sold in high street shops, they are amongst the smaller end of the fat spectrum, and this does not necessarily mean that there is also a huge population of women who wear a size 30/32/34 and above.

This numbers game has had an impact on relations between fat people. Smaller fat people may believe that their perspective is the most correct since it is more common, whilst super-sized people's claims on fat rights continue to be dismissed. For example, Caroline Currey points out that within some anti-diet rhetoric:

> There's usually a cut-off point. It's like: 'We will agree with the set point theory up to 15 stone' and over 15 stone suddenly people are supposed to be something else, and then dieting is recommended, and stomach stapling, and all the rest of that sort of garbage.

I believe that unless size rights issues are applicable to all fat people, then the arguments in favour of, for example, set point theory, are worthless. Furthermore, these divisions feed beliefs about fat people who are acceptable, and those who are not. Viv Wachenje remarks:

> I do have to say that I don't find gross obesity attractive, that's my honest opinion. I'm talking about people who have got to about 40 stone; I don't find that attractive. Generally I like the variety of shape, of contour. I'm not anti-slim people either. People's shapes are important, they're a turn-on, but I do have my own prejudice, and

gross obesity I don't find attractive. I find I gawp in horror.

Whilst taste and prejudice are moot points, I question the value of supporting divisive arguments which encourage very fat people to be targeted in this way, especially within the context of a movement which seeks to free everyone from body hatred.

So within the fat rights movement who is free from discrimination? Not thinner people, not smaller fat people, not people who suffer eating disorders and not super-sized people. All must deal with exclusion. To me this means that the movement has not yet come to terms with the notion of difference, and that in many areas it still adopts a good/bad dualism with regard to different degrees of fatness, rather than a thorough celebration of all body sizes. It also suggests that some factions within the movement are developing new standards of 'normality', rather than abandoning such standards altogether, and these are creating new patterns of exclusion and domination based on ignorance and mistrust. I hope that we can begin to challenge our prejudice, and to destroy the divisive contingents of 'them' and 'us'.

Fat Admirers

Fat Admirers (FAS) are people, often thinner men, who have a particular sexual interest in fat people, most often fat women. Fat Admirer is the preferred self-definition, but FAS are sometimes also known as 'chubby chasers'. Some FAS seek to define their interest in fat people as a sexual identity, others consider it a political affiliation. As a socially marginalised group, there is a stigma attached to people who find us attractive, but those people consider FA relationships as an ideal match between two interested parties. In the US, FAS exercise power and influence in the size rights movement in a variety of areas; for example, NAAFA's founder is an FA, there are FAS on the boards of various fat rights organisations, whilst others can be found at many social gatherings.

Some people consider their attraction to fat people a fetish. Many fat people find this offensive because it is seen to negate one's humanity and individuality. Others find the idea of people being attracted to us *because* we are fat highly seductive and to be enjoyed. Sometimes this has positive repercussions for our self-esteem, as Mandy found out:

> It was really through Richard, my ex-boyfriend, who was really the first guy I'd ever met in my life that was into big women, that I trusted, that I knew for real that he wasn't going to take the piss. It was through him really that I became proud within myself.

Most of us live in societies where fat bodies are seen as ugly and undesirable, so fetishising fatness can be very sexy to fat people when negative cultural messages are reversed, and one's body becomes highly valued.

Fat Admirers present many conflicts for feminists, and contradict classic feminist theory about the purpose and meaning of women's body fat. In *Fat is a Feminist Issue* Orbach argues that women gain weight intentionally yet subconsciously to avoid having to deal with emotions surrounding our sexuality. Far from being asexual, FAS show that fat can be considered hyper-sexual. Moreover, Orbach's vision of fat women's sexuality is defined in terms of 'pressure', of us being helpless victims of men. I find this a patronising analysis which is out of touch with the reality of women's sexuality.

FA relationships are also under suspicion as destructive and abusive. In cultures where women's independence is regarded as threatening, we experience many social pressures to find a husband or a partner. Perhaps we have not had a chance as fat people to express our needs or desires concerning relationships, we may feel vulnerable and inhibited by fat hatred. Low self-esteem, cultural pressures and fantasies surrounding love and romance, plus the confusion we might feel about our sexuality as fat people, all contribute to making us vulnerable to relationships where we are not equals, and where there is abuse and dependence. We might also feel that relationships like these are all we can expect.

I am not suggesting that all relationships between fat people and FAS are questionable, but the emphasis on appearance over substance is suspect. I am concerned that FAS fetishise our bodies regardless of our consent, believing, for example, that our fatness makes us more feminine, more beautiful, more nurturing, or more dependent than anybody else. Is this stereotyping any different from that practised by individuals who are only attracted to thinner people, or women with large breasts? When fat people are treated as trophies we are stripped of our humanity. It implies that we are no longer considered to be whole, thinking, feeling people. Some FA relationships seem to offer safety from the hostility that is often directed towards our fat bodies, but being the object of chivalry and protection is stifling, it fosters dependency and prevents us from developing for ourselves. Furthermore it is patronising, it implies that FAS are more able to cope than we are, and in a better position to protect us.

Another bone of contention is that some fat rights organisations depend on FAS, either financially or as a carrot on a stick to attract new members, and some fat activist organisations, such as *Rump Parliament*, include FAS as allies. Other organisations do not, for the reasons I have outlined above among others. Some FAS insist that they are not tolerated because fat people cannot bear any sexual attention to be drawn to our bodies, which fits with Orbach's argument about women using the fat on our bodies as a means of hiding from our sexuality. I think that it is unfair to assume that all fat people should feel the same way, and this position also presumes that we should always be ready and grateful for FA attention! More seriously, these beliefs demean us by continually treating fat people as potential conquests whether or not we want this.

I believe that a person does not have to be fat in order to be a fat activist, although fat people currently have a personal interest in ending fat hatred. However, FAS have a different agenda from activists, and this is another source of conflict. In a personal communication, Karen W Stimson asserts:

I don't want to come across as a separatist of any stripe here, but I do think that the fact that FAS have a different agenda from those they 'admire', the high (perceived) ratio of available fat women to male FAS, and the power of patriarchy in general, among other things, combines to make abuse almost inevitable when we give thin male FAS the power to determine or represent fat women's best interests.

In theory fat activist and FA need not be mutually exclusive labels, but this does not always work in practice. Karen continues:

When I wrote you that 'fat admirers who do not exploit and are politically aware' can be allies of fat people, it was a statement more based on solidarity theory than reality, because I don't personally know any non-fat FAS who don't exploit or abuse fat women. At least I can't think of any right now.

Whether or not an FA is exploitative may depend on whether or not they themselves are fat. Thinner FAS might not have as deep an understanding of fat issues as do FAS who are fat. But being fat does not preclude an individual from being abusive themselves. Karen adds:

There are a lot of equally slimy fat male FAS – one of them is poisoning an e-mail list we are on right now. But they're not in positions of authority in the movement as the thin FAS are, partly because of the prejudice of many fat women against fat men as sexual partners. This points up the complicity fat women have in creating or perpetuating abuse.

It seems that there are many conflicts for feminists, fat activists and FAs to resolve, such as consent, mutual respect and an understanding of fat politics.

All Together Now?

I have misgivings about criticising the size rights movement so publicly since fat people are not organising from a position of social power and status, and fat activists are already being maligned. Read, for example, columnist Zoe Heller's comments about 'Fat Libbers' who 'complain about how beautiful – how healthy – fat is'. She continues:

> Everyone knows they are on to a loser, and yet the talk shows keep bringing them back, again and again, to jiggle about in their kaftans insisting that slimness is actually revolting and that morbid obesity can be a very sexy lifestyle option.[3]

With public support like this I have no desire to exacerbate the problems between competing factions, or create new witch-hunts within the movement. Other groups are already experiencing a hardening of attitudes from a backlash against political correctness, and this is filtering into fat politics. The early fat rights movement, such as the Fat Underground, and the first London Fat Women's Group, had strong ties with radical lesbian feminists, presented by many critics as arch-proponents of pc: dogmatic, unrelenting and out of touch with ordinary lives.

As fat people become more organised and uppity, we should bear in mind that there are people and organisations who have profits and status to lose by our empowerment. There are groups who will resent our power and influence, for example, business owners may regard the expense and effort of implementing size-positive legislation as arduous and unreasonable. In seeking equality, respect and acceptance, fat people are challenging fundamental institutions which promote bedrock beliefs about health and normality. Consequently, I believe that there will be no social change without a struggle.

Like the fat rights movement, the dieting industry is not a monolithic entity. Diet proponents are often in competition with each other to capture the market. Weight-loss advocates cover a broad range of interests which are not necessarily related – for example manufacturers of diet drinks, commercial weight-loss support groups, and publishers of dieting magazines and books are all separate industries which have only their support of fat hatred in common. Therefore the backlash from these industries will occur on a variety of fronts. Moreover, these industries will use any scam they can to sell their products and ideas, as long as they tie in with contemporary fantasies, or beliefs. There is nothing to stop them from incorporating non-diet ideas into their sales pitch without altering the content of their product or service. Hence 'dieting' becomes transformed into 'healthy eating plans'. Caroline Currey expands:

> The anti-diet movement is becoming quite popular, and there is a rise of anti-diet organisations. Even Weight Watchers is now, I think, 'anti-diet'. I wonder do they still clap when you lose weight? Or is it a sort of silent approval? There is a switch to 'healthy eating' and 'good' exercise regimes, but really as long as fatness is seen as bad, none of the problems are going to go away.

On a personal level many of our friends and acquaintances feel threatened when fat people begin to make demands. Discussing a fat ex-lover, one woman comments:

> She impressed upon me how much more oppressed than

me, being fat, she was, and that I was at fault, because my vision was twisted by patriarchal values of beauty, currently thin.[4]

To such people it must seem as though we have suddenly moved the goalposts and set impossible new rules. Elana Dykewomon records one woman's response to fat rights issues as 'Is this the new thing we have to be pc about?'[5] In this context there is a temptation for the threatened party to dismiss fat politics as tangential, and less legitimate when compared to 'real' oppression. Dykewomon remarks of fat politics that it:

> still doesn't qualify as real political thought, it's viewed as a leisure pursuit of the bourgeoise [sic] who want to be left alone to be self-indulgent in peace; or that it's 'cashing in' on the political groundwork done by other groups (even if fat womyn are members of 'other groups').

I believe that all people must take some responsibility in order to challenge prejudice, but I think fat people should be wary of enforcing new patterns of guilt when we point the finger, as this encourages people to respond to fat politics with defensiveness, denial and anger.

I have chosen to criticise some aspects of size rights publicly because I believe that silence will not resolve problems within the movement. I also believe that constructive criticism leads to a flowering of growth and development. If the fat rights movement wants to achieve a lasting and deep social change in favour of fat people, then it needs to be strong and agile, it must create watertight responses to the inevitable backlashes. I hope that my criticisms will help build a firmer base on which to develop new ideas about fat rights. However, in many ways the size rights movement already enjoys a solid foundation and, for me, the positive attributes of the fat rights community will always far outweigh the negative.

Conclusion
No Turning Back

What motivates fat people and the fat rights movement is a righteous anger at injustice and abuse, but also the hope that we can effect a positive change. Unlike the systems we criticise such as dieting industries and medicine, the movement is not mobilised by money or status, but exists for the common good. Our potential for power is exciting. Caroline Currey comments:

It feels like our time is coming. It feels like an idea is just about to be realised.

Many of us bring utopian visions to our activism, like Max Airborne:

> I want a world where fat is beautiful, of course. I want everyone to love themselves. I want the diet industry to crash because nobody is obsessed with losing weight any more. I want to walk into any clothing store and find clothes to fit me. I want couches in movie theatres. I want to walk down the street and be respected instead of ridiculed.

As fat activists we seek practical ways to transform our dreams into reality. Given the cultural context of fat hatred and shame, our hope in the future is truly moving and inspirational.

The fat rights movement is political. We follow the tradition of other groups struggling for civil rights. Fat politics makes sense of fat oppression by setting the personal and private world within a political context. The fat rights movement embraces what has come to be known as identity politics, which asserts the right of an oppressed group to define and challenge the source of their oppression. As such it is managed by fat people because we are the only group who are truly qualified to speak out for ourselves. This is an empowering departure from the medical models, which define fat people as sick and abnormal, and which encourage us to feel ashamed and embarrassed about our bodies.

The fat rights movement is accessible. It is based on the reality of our experiences and feelings, not the fantasy of another weight-loss diet. Size acceptance is achievable by everyone, unlike the lies promoted as aspirations by weight-loss proponents. Within the movement people who, elsewhere, are often forced into marginal social roles here take centre stage. It is a movement where women are the driving force for change, from Fat Lip Readers Theatre, to the Fat Women's Group and beyond. I am also personally proud to say that lesbians, such as the members of the Fat Underground have consistently provided a biting and innovative commentary on fat oppression within the movement. More recently the DIY culture of zines, support groups and internet resources, rather than large organisations, are offering a new dynamic approach to fat rights issues.

There has been no overnight revolution. Dieting and weight-loss cures are marketed as a quick and accessible fix for a variety of chronic problems, from loneliness to fears of ill-health and low self-esteem. When fat people relinquish weight-loss fantasies our problems often remain, and many of us come to fat politics seeking a fast solution. It is depressing to find that there is no instant answer, and that long-term difficulties require an extended commitment if they are to be disentangled. People lose hope that anything will ever change, but change on the scale we desire does not happen quickly. Nevertheless people have been campaigning around fat rights issues for nearly thirty years, and over that period some massive transformations have been achieved.

Fat people's intolerance of fat hatred has filtered into the outside world. Attitudes towards fat people have altered enough that, for example, the climate will support a book such as this. Businesses are beginning to take account of our needs, especially in areas such as clothing, and service providers, such as the media, are beginning to acknowledge our ideas. Fat people are beginning to take legal action against harassment and abuse, and anti-diet legislation is now a possibility. There have even been changes amongst health professionals' attitudes to fat people although, given the weight of medical fatphobia, these have been very small, and with many conditions attached.

Fat people have created a multifaceted movement. We have even invented a language with which to identify concepts such as size acceptance and fat hatred. As a community our history of struggle and resistance is impressive, and our support networks, activists, coalitions, magazines and organisations continue to bring us together and fight for our rights.

One of the most important changes has been the shift taking place within our own heads, how we understand ourselves and our relationship to the rest of the world. For many people personal empowerment is a prime reason for one's involvement with the fat rights movement. Jean Midson explains:

> If I can express and show that I'm okay with me that's probably the most important thing.

Fat politics enables us to generate better self-esteem without weight loss being a condition. Personal empowerment has allowed many of us to become our own role models, and to live without the disabling feelings of shame and embarrassment towards our bodies. Feeling good about ourselves has also helped us to connect with other fat people, and to appreciate what it means to be fat. Max Airborne contends:

> I am finding fat women really sexy, way more than I did before. I think this comes from liking myself and my body more.

Fat people have begun to think about our bodies in a different way, one which enables us to question our classification as diseased pariahs, and develop new debates and ideas. We are learning that as fat people we do not have to put up with fat hatred.

Thirty years ago, a period that is around my lifetime, there was silence.

The Interview Sample

I am very grateful to the women in the sample for giving their time and commitment to this book. What follows are some brief biographical notes, which I include so that readers will have more of an idea of the context in which the quotations were made.

Max Airborne
I'm a 29-year-old fat dyke. I've been fat since I was a kid, though looking back I see that I was never as fat as I was

made to feel by my family and other kids. I began the long process of accepting my body after I came out as a young teenager and started thinking politically. I had previously been on forced diets since a very young age and was kept in a psychiatric hospital for a year and a half (age thirteen–fifteen) on a 50-calorie-a-day diet. Even after I was released I had to travel by train 200 miles round trip two or three times a week to 'weigh in', with the constant threat of being locked up again. Now I am part of a collective that publishes a magazine for fat dykes called *FaT GiRL*. We try to integrate discussion about fat issues with dyke issues and dyke sexuality.

Annette Cooper
I've taken early retirement from my job as a trainer for British Telecom, 45-years old. Don't need to earn money so I'm looking for purpose and fulfilment. Big crossroads for me.

Caroline Currey
I'm 43, and I'm a naturally fat woman who tried to keep her weight down with eating disorders.

Ellen
I am 38, a professional office administrator and volunteer literacy tutor. I am married, with no children, and live in a city on the West Coast of the United States. I am American and lived in Britain for eight years.

Janne
I'm 26 and I'm black. I was born in this country and I've lived round here [London] for about two years. I'm bisexual since about October last year.

Kristine Kay
I'm 38-years-old and I've lived in the UK since 1981. I have a bachelor's degree in Mass Communications, I work as a caretaker in a block of flats, and I'm studying for my City

and Guilds in embroidery. Oh yes, I come from a very large family.

Lee Kennedy
I'm a mega-fat person, I work in a slave job, and I'm a cartoonist and writer.

Lucy
I'm a white able-bodied, fat Sagittarian lesbian. Currently 27 (but generally feeling about 112)!

Mandy
I'm a fabulous, gorgeous, lovely woman and I love myself most of the time.

Jean Midson
I live on my own apart from two cats. I've been here eleven years in Harlow, and I like it very much.

Karen W Stimson
Co-director of Largesse, the Network for Size Esteem (with my husband Richard). I've been fat all my life and a fat activist for over half of it. I am an artist, writer and designer.

Viv Wachenje
I've lived in Harlow ever since I was three. I've always been regarded as plump, or sturdy, or well-built.

Yvette Williams Elliott
I work as a lecturer part time at the University of East London, where I'm also doing my PhD, hopefully around issues related to fat. I think of myself as a very fat woman.

Notes

Introduction

1   Susie Orbach, *Fat is a Feminist Issue*, Arrow, London, 1978

2   L Schoenfielder and B Wieser, *Shadow on a Tightrope: Writings by Women on Fat Oppression*, Aunt Lute, Iowa, 1983; Rotunda, Glasgow, 1989. Shelley Bovey, *Being Fat is not a Sin*, Pandora, London, 1989

3   Robin Tolmach Lakoff and Raquel Scherr, *Face Value: The Politics of Beauty*, Routledge and Kegan Paul, Boston, 1984, p 248

4   See, for example, Wendy Chapkis, *Beauty Secrets: Women and the Politics of Appearance*, The Women's Press, London, 1986; and Rita Freedman, *Beauty Bound: Why Women Strive for Physical Perfection*, Columbus, London, 1990

5   Naomi Wolf, *The Beauty Myth: How Images of Beauty are Used Against Women*, Chatto & Windus, London, 1990

6   Chapkis, op. cit., p 32

7   Nicky Diamond, 'Thin is the Feminist Issue', *Feminist Review* 19, Spring, 1995

8   Freedman, op. cit., p 153

9   Diamond, op. cit, p 49

10 Orland W Wooley and Susan C Wooley, 'Obesity and Women I – A Closer Look at the Facts and Obesity' and 'Obesity and Women II – A Neglected Feminist Topic', *Women's Studies International Quarterly* vol. 2, 1979

11 Kelly, 'The Goddess is Fat' in Schoenfielder and Wieser, op. cit., pp 15–21

Chapter One: Identifying Fatphobia

1   R Howe, 'Style Directors', *ES Magazine*, 30 September 1994

2   P Platt, 'The Fat Busters', *Guardian*, 16 November 1993

3   Victor Lewis Smith, 'As Advertised by Hugh Grant', *Evening Standard*, 7 July 1995

4   Alison Pearson, 'Comic Oprah from Weighty Issues', *Observer Review*, 24 September 1995

5   Germaine Greer, 'Obscenity of the Finger Food Feasters', *Guardian*, 6 October 1994

6   Tina Ogle, 'Fat of the Land', *Time Out*, 9 December 1992

7   Joan Dickenson, 'Some Thoughts on Fat' in Schoenfielder and Wieser, op. cit., p 48

8   Stevens, Kumanyika, and Keil, cited in Diane Adams, *Health Issues for Women of Colour: A Cultural Diversity Perspective*, Sage, London/California, 1995, pp 117–18

9   Donna Allegra, 'Fat Dancer' in Carol Wiley, *Journeys to Self-Acceptance: Fat Women Speak*, The Crossing Press, California, 1994, p 109

10   Sondra Solovay, 'the good, the bad . . . and the indigestible', *Fat!So?* #3, 1995, p 14

11   Donald Bogle, *Toms, Coons, Mulattoes, Mammies & Bucks: An Interpretive History of Blacks in American Films*, Roundhouse, Oxford, 1994

12   Allegra, op. cit., pp 108–9

13   Dickenson, op., cit., p 46

14   Valerie Mason-John, 'Keeping up Appearances: The Body and Eating Habits' in N Godwin, B Hollows and S. Nye, *Assaults on Convention: Essays on Lesbian Transgressors*, Cassell, London, 1996, p 76

15   Anna Johnson, 'Anna's Place', *Living Large*, September/October 1996

16   Honorine Woodward, 'the fatter adventures of super-mom #9', *Living Large*, January/February 1997

17   Allegra, op. cit., p 109

Chapter Two: Responding to Fatphobia

1   Rosemary Green, *Diary of a Fat Housewife: A True Story of Humour, Heartbreak and Hope*, Warner Books, New York, 1995

Chapter Three: Living Fat

No Notes

Chapter Four: Danger! Obesity!

1   Susan Sontag, *Illness as a Metaphor*, Penguin, London, 1977

2   Richard Klein, *Eat Fat*, Picador, London, 1997

3   Royal College of Physicians, *Obesity*, RCP, London, 1983

4   Wooley and Wooley, op. cit.

5   Paul Ernsberger and Paul Haskew, 'Rethinking Obesity: An Alternative View of its Health Implications' in *Journal of Obesity and Weight Regulation*, vol. 6 #2 Summer, Human Science Press, New York, 1987
6   Stephen Mennell, 'On the Civilising of Appetite' in M. Featherstone, M Hepworth, and B S Turner. *The Body: Social Process and Cultural Theory*, Sage, London, 1991, p 150
7   Klein, op. cit., p 103
8   Margaret Greaves, *Big and Beautiful: Challenging the Myths and Celebrating our Size*, Grafton, London, 1990
9   H Canning and J Muir, 'Obesity – Its Possible Effects on College Acceptance,' *New England Journal of Medicine*, vol. 275, 1966

Chapter Five: Eating Disorders and Red Herrings

1   Eating Disorders Association information leaflet
2   Orbach, *Fat is a Feminist Issue*, op. cit. and Susie Orbach, *Fat is Feminist Issue 2*, Hamlyn, London, 1982. Kim Chernin, *Womansize: The Tyranny of Slenderness*, The Women's Press, London, 1981
3   Orbach, *Fat is a Feminist Issue*, op. cit., p 18
4   Ibid., p 39
5   Chernin, *Womansize*, op. cit., p 73
6   Ibid., p 80
7   Orbach, *Fat is a Feminist Issue 2*, op. cit., pp 11–12
8   Ibid., p 12
9   Chernin, *Womansize*, op. cit., p 86
10 Orbach, *Fat is a Feminist Issue*, op. cit., p 35
11 Susie Orbach, *Hunger Strike: The Anorectic's Struggle as a Metaphor of our Age*, Faber & Faber, London, 1986
12 Kim Chernin, *The Hungry Self: Women, Eating, and Identity*, Virago, London, 1986
13 Jo Ind, *Fat is a Spiritual Issue: My Journey*, Mowbray, London, 1993. Irene O'Garden, *Fat Girl: One Woman's Way Out*, HarperCollins, New York, 1993

14 bell hooks, *Sisters of the Yam: Black Women and Self-Recovery*, Turnaround, London, 1993
15 Mason-John, op. cit.
16 Susan Powter, *Stop the Insanity!*, Orion, London, 1994
17 R M Meadow and L Weiss, *Women's Conflicts about Eating and Sexuality: The Relationship Between Food and Sex*, The Haworth Press, Boston, 1992
18 Sue Dyson, *A Weight Off Your Mind. How to Stop Worrying about Your Body Size*, Sheldon Press, London, 1991
19 Shelley Bovey, *The Forbidden Body*, Pandora, London, 1994
20 Wiley, op. cit.

Chapter Six: Cures

1 National Institutes of Health, 1992
2 Klein, op. cit.
3 Mary Evans Young, *Dietbreaking: Having it All Without Having to Diet*, Hodder & Stoughton, London, 1995, p 78
4 Charlotte Cooper, *The Fear of Fat: An Investigation into the Politics of Size Acceptance*, University of East London, 1994, p 38
5 Susan C Wooley, 'Psychological and Social Aspects of Obesity', in A E Bender and L B Brooks (eds), *Body Weight Control; The Physiology, Clinical Treatment, and Prevention of Obesity*, Churchill Livingstone, London, 1991
6 Ernsberger and Haskew, op. cit., p 48
7 Kathy O'Donnell, 'Why I Had My Stomach Stapled', *Me*, 10 August 1992
8 Susan C Wooley, op. cit., p 87
9 Ernsberger and Haskew, op. cit.
10 Susan C Wooley, op. cit., p 82
11 Cooper, *The Fear of Fat*, p 21
12 A Hernandez, 'Judy FreeSpirit', *FatGirl#1*, 1994
13 Karen W Stimson, *Size Rights: The Disability Debate*, Largesse, Connecticut, 1994

14 Carrie Hemenway, 'Dispelling Common Myths about Fat People', NAAFA information leaflet

Chapter Seven: Fat Rights History

1   Llewellyn Louderback, *Fat Power: Thin May Be In, But Fat's Where It's At!*, Hawthorne Books, Boston, 1970
2   Alice Ansfield and L Cunkle, 'All Set to Fight Discrimination', *Radiance*, Spring 1989
3   NAAFA press pack
4   Karen Smith, 'Space', *Living Large*, September/October, 1995
5   Louderback, op. cit.
6   Karen W Stimson, *The Fat Underground*, Largesse, Connecticut, 1994
7   Ibid.
8   Ansfield and Cunkle, op. cit.
9   Karen W Stimson, *Fat Feminist Herstory*, Largesse, Connecticut, 1994
10 C Currey, 'Books We Have Loved' in Charlotte Cooper, *A Fat Woman's Resource Directory*, The Fat Women's Group, London, 1995
11 Cooper, *The Fear of Fat*, op. cit., p 55
12 Tina Jenkins and Margaret Farnham, 'As I Am', *Trouble and Strife* 13, Spring, 1988
13 Heather Smith 'Creating a Politics of Appearance', *Trouble and Strife* 16, Summer, 1989
14 Bovey, *Being Fat is not a Sin*, op. cit., p 9
15 Bovey, *The Forbidden Body*, op. cit., pp 257–8

Chapter Eight: The Fat Rights Movement Today

1   Wooley and Wooley, op. cit.
2   Ernsberger and Haskew, op. cit.
3   Hillel Schwartz, *Never Satisfied: A Cultural History of Diets, Fantasies, and Fat*, The Free Press, New York, 1986
4   Laura Brown and Esther D Rothblum, *Overcoming*

Fear of Fat (also published as *Fat Oppression and Psythotherapy: A Feminist Perspective*), The Haworth Press, Boston, 1989

5 See Jane Ogden. *Fat Chance! The Myth of Dieting Explained*, Routledge, London, 1992

6 Pat Lyons and Debby Burgard, *Great Shape: The First Fitness Guide for Large Women*, Bull Publishing Company, Palo Alto, California, 1990

7 Large and Lovely Club information sheet.

8 Susan Stinson, *Fat Girl Dances with Rocks*, Spinster's Ink, Minneapolis, 1994; *Martha Moody*, The Women's Press, London, 1996

9 Laurie Toby Edison and Debbie Notkin, *Women En Large: Images of Fat Nudes*, Books in Focus, San Francisco, 1994

10 R Field and C Jackson, 'Broadening Out', *Trouble and Strife* 23, Spring, 1992

11 Seth Friedman, 'Editorial', *Factsheet* 5#57, August, 1995

12 M Wann, 'Fat!So? Manifesto', *Fat!So?* #2, 1994

Chapter Nine: All Together Now?

1 Dyson, op.cit., p 34

2 Karis Otobong, 'Fattened by Force', *Trouble and Strife* 23, Spring, 1992

3 Zoe Heller, 'Home Thoughts from the Land of Excess', *Independent on Sunday*, 20 August 1994

4 M King, 'It Can't be Either' in S Rose, C Stevens *et al*, *Bisexual Horizons: Politics Histories Lives*, Laurence & Wishart, London, 1995

5 Elana Dykewomon, 'Travelling Fat', in Schoenfielder and Wieser, op.cit., p 150

Conclusion
No Notes

Resources

This is not a complete list of every fat rights resource in the world, although I have tried to feature as many British organisations as possible. Some of the initiatives listed here are mentioned in this book, some are not, but all provide a good jumping-in point for those interested in size rights issues. Most of these resources operate on very small budgets, especially the zines, so if you write please enclose a stamped addressed envelope, International Reply Coupons, money or stamps to cover postage.

Activist Organisations

Association For The Health Enrichment of Large People (AHELP)
PO Drawer C, Radford, VA 24143, USA
tel: 00 1 800 368 3468 x 501

Body Image Task Force
PO Box 934, Santa Cruz, CA 95061-0934, USA
tel: 00 1 408 457 4838
e-mail: datkins@blue.weeg.uiowa.edu

Council on Size and Weight Discrimination Inc.
PO Box 305, Mount Marion, NY 12456, USA
tel: 00 1 914 679 1209

Largesse
PO Box 9404, New Haven, CT 06534-0404, USA
tel/fax: 00 1 207 787 1624
e-mail: 75773.717@compuserve.com

National Association to Advance Fat Acceptance (NAAFA)
PO Box 188620, Sacramento, CA 95818, USA
tel: 00 1 916 558 6880
fax: 00 1 916 558 6881
Contact NAAFA for address details of its Special Interest Groups and local chapters.

NAAFA Fat Feminist Caucus
c/o Judy Freespirit, 407 Orange Street #101, Oakland, CA 94610, USA

Rump Parliament
PO Box 181716, Dallas, TX 75218, USA
tel: 00 1 214 275 4449
e-mail: 72113.2500@compuserve.com

SIZE
c/o Diana Pollard, Ten Palace Gate, London W8 5NF
tel/fax: 0171 700 0509
e-mail: dwm@premier.co.uk

Size Acceptance Network
c/o Dion Zuess, Size Acceptance Network Coordinator,
Eastern Community Health Service, Box 5, 5 Darley Road,
Paradise, SA 5075, Australia
tel: 00 61 08 207 8933
fax: 00 61 08 365 2223

Commercial Products and Services

Amplestuff Ltd.
PO Box 116, Bearsville, NY 12409, USA
tel: 00 1 914 679 3316
fax: 00 1 914 679 1209

Bulk
A nightclub for fat gay men and their admirers. The venue
has changed several times. At the time of writing it takes
place on Saturdays at Club 180, 180 Earls Court Road,
London W5, but check the gay press to be sure, or e-mail
bobby@powerhouse.co.uk

Chubby Companions
21 Ulundi Street, Radcliffe, Greater Manchester M26 3AN
tel: 0161 724 6791

Le Grand Weekend
38 Westbury Lodge Close, Pinner, Middlesex HA5 3FG
tel: 0181 933 2091

Miss Big and Beautiful
tel: 0181 870 0624

Planet Big Girl
PO Box 4110, London SE15 4LR
tel: 0171 639 0914

Plump Partners
8 Sealand Avenue, Holywell, Clwyd CH8 7BU
tel: 01352 715909

Royal Resources
PO Box 220, Camas Valley, OR 97416, USA
tel: 00 1 503 445 2330

Rubenesque Romances
PO Box 534, Tarrytown, NY 10591-0534, USA

Exercise Groups

Big Aerobics for Big People
158 Westbury Avenue, London N22 6RT
tel: 0181 888 0569

Big in Fitness
9 Anzio Crescent, Lincoln LN1 3PS
tel: 01522 569148

Fat and Fit
c/o Health Action, 1 Pink Lane, Newcastle-upon-Tyne
NE1 5DW

Internet

Try the *Fat!So?* page on the World Wide Web for links to
other fat-positive web sites. Two newsgroups to start off
with are: alt.support.big-folks, and soc.support.fat-
acceptance. All are good places to find out about other
newsgroups and e-mail lists.

Magazines

Big Beautiful Woman
LFP Inc., 9171 Wilshire Boulevard, Beverly Hills, CA 90210, USA

Dimensions
PO Box 640, Folsom, CA 95763-0640, USA
tel: 00 1 916 984 9447

Extra! Magazine
PO Box 57194, Sherman Oaks, CA 91413, USA
tel: 00 1 818 997 8404
fax: 00 1 818 909 0758

Radiance: The Magazine for Large Women
PO Box 30246, Oakland, CA 94604, USA
tel/fax: 00 1 510 482 0680
e-mail: radmag@aol.com

Yes!
90 Banner Street, London EC1Y 8JU
tel: 0171 608 3664

Non-Diet Initiatives

Abundia
4921 Whiffin Place, Downer's Grove, IL 60515, USA
tel: 00 1 818 997 8404

Dietbreakers/Mary Evans Young
Church Cottage, Barford St Michael, Banbury, Oxon OX15 0UA
tel: 01869 337070
fax: 01869 337177

Eating Disorders Association
Sackville Place, 44 Magdalen Street, Norwich, Norfolk NR3 1JU
tel: 01603 621414

Women, Food and Feelings
Community and Leisure, Harlow Council, Latton Bush Centre, Southern Way, Harlow, Essex CM18 7BL

You*Nique
620 Jarvis Street, Suite 1023, Toronto, Ontario M4Y 2R8, Canada
tel: 00 1 416 964 0292
e-mail: younique@ablelink.org

Support Groups

Allegro Fortissimo
26 rue de la Vega, 75012 Paris, France

Bond van Formaat
PO Box 216, 5500 AE Veldhoven, The Netherlands
fax: 00 31 36 53 66 975
e-mail: obistat@via.nl, with either Bond van Formaat or Society of Size as subject.

Dicke.e.V.
PO Box 410105, 34063 Kassel, Germany
fax: 00 49 561 39018

Fat is a Lesbian Issue and
Fat Lesbian Action Brigade (FLAB)
c/o Gail Horowitz and Shira Stone, 225C King Street, Princeton, NJ 08540, USA
tel: 00 1 609 924 9321
e-mail: sestone@ponyexpress.princeton.edu

The Fat Women's Group
The WHEEL, 4 Wild Court, London WC2B 5AU

Lesbian Fat Activist Network
PO Box 635, Woodstock, NY 12498, USA
tel: 00 1 914 679 9019
e-mail: 76473.2141@compuserve.com

SAFFIR
4649 Sunnyside Avenue North Room #222, Seattle, WA
98103, USA

SAFFO
c/o UYW, 244 Coffman Union, 300 Washington Ave. SE,
Minneapolis, MN 55455, USA

Sisters of Size
710 28th Avenue South, Seattle, WA 98114, USA

WOW – Women of Width
e-mail: jwermont@netcom.com

Theatre

4 Big Girls
343¹/₂ 17th Avenue, Seattle, WA 98122-5706, USA
tel: 00 1 206 323 5171

Fat Lip Readers Theatre
PO Box 29963, Oakland, CA 94604, USA

Zines

Fat!So?
PO Box 423464, San Francisco, CA 94142, USA
e-mail: Marilynwann@pop.sirius.com

Girlfrenzy #4 The Fat Liberation Issue
PO Box 148, Hove, East Sussex BN3 3DQ

i'm so fucking beautiful
c/o 120 State NE#1510, Olympia, WA 98501, USA

Lee Kennedy Comics
58 Durrington Tower, Westbury, Wandsworth Road, London SW8 3LF

Living Large
Box 439, Lisle, IL 60532-0439, USA
e-mail: Cadyem@aol.com

Lone Star Comics
Flat 10, 24 Park Crescent, Brighton BN2 3HA

Red Hanky Panky
7 Old School Buildings, St Clements Yard, Archdown Road, London SE22 9HP

Bibliography

Adams, D L, *Health Issues for Women of Colour: A Cultural Diversity Perspective* Sage, California/London, 1995

Allegra, D, 'Fat Dancer' in C Wiley, *Journeys To Self-Acceptance: Fat Women Speak*, The Crossing Press, California, 1994

Ansfield, A and L Cunkle, 'All Set To Fight Discrimination', *Radiance: The Magazine for Large Women*, Spring 1989

Ashworth, S, *A Matter of Fat*, Crocus/Commonword Ltd

Signet, Manchester, London, 1991/1993

Bogle, D, *Toms, Coons, Mulattoes, Mammies & Bucks: An Interpretive History of Blacks in American Films*, Roundhouse, Oxford, 1994

Bornstein, K, *Gender Outlaw: On Men, Women and the Rest of Us*, Routledge, New York, 1994

Bovey, S, *Being Fat is not a Sin*, Pandora, London, 1989
—*The Forbidden Body*, Pandora, London, 1994

Brown, L S and E Rothblum, *Overcoming Fear of Fat* (also published as *Fat Oppression and Psychotherapy: A Feminist Perspective*, The Haworth Press, Boston 1989

Califia, P, "Big Girls", *Melting Point*, Alyson Publications, Boston, 1993

Canning, H and J Muir, 'Obesity – Its Possible Effects on College Acceptance', *New England Journal of Medicine*, vol. 275, 1966

Caskey, N, 'Interpreting Anorexia Nervosa' in S R Suleiman, *The Female Body in Western Culture: Contemporary Perspectives*, Harvard University Press, Boston, 1985

Chapkis, W, *Beauty Secrets: Women and the Politics of Appearance*, London, The Women's Press, 1986

Chernin, K, *Womansize: The Tyranny of Slenderness*, The Women's Press, London, 1986
— *The Hungry Self: Women, Eating and Identity*, Virago, London, 1986

Christine, 'Heavy SM: Fat Brats Speak Out', *BratAttack* #1, 1991

Cooper, C, *The Fear of Fat: An Investigation into the Politics of Size Acceptance*, University of East London, 1994

Coupland, D, 'Brentwood Notebook', *Polaroids From the Dead*, HarperCollins, New York, 1996

Currey, C, 'Books We Have Loved', in C Cooper, *A Fat Woman's Resource Directory*, London, The Fat Women's Group, London, 1995

Davis, K, *Reshaping the Female Body: The Dilemma of*

Cosmetic Surgery, Routledge, London, 1995

Diamond, N, 'Thin is the Feminist Issue', *Feminist Review* 19, Spring 1995

Dickenson, J, 'Some Thoughts on Fat', in *Shadow on a Tightrope* (see Schoenfielder L and B Wieser)

Dykewomon, E, 'Travelling Fat', *Shadow on a Tightrope* (see Schoenfielder L and B Wieser)

Dyson, S, *A Weight Off Your Mind: How to Stop Worrying About Your Body Size*, Sheldon Press, London, 1991

Edison, L T, and D Notkin, *Women En Large: Images of Fat Nudes*, Books In Focus, San Francisco, 1994

Ernsberger, P and P Haskew, 'Rethinking Obesity: An Alternative View of its Health Implications', *The Journal of Obesity and Weight Regulation* vol. 6 #2, *Human Science Press*, 1987

Evans Young, M, *Dietbreaking: Having It All Without Having to Diet*, Hodder & Stoughton, London, 1995

Feinberg, L, *Stone Butch Blues*, Firebrand, New York, 1993

Field, R and C Jackson, 'Broadening Out', *Trouble and Strife* 23, Spring 1992

Freedman, R, *Beauty Bound: Why Women Strive for Physical Perfection*, Columbus, London, 1988

Friedman, 'Editorial', *Factsheet* 5 #57, August 1995

Greaves, M, *Big and Beautiful: Challenging the Myths and Celebrating Our Size*, Grafton London, 1990

Green, R, *Diary of a Fat Housewife: A True Story of Humour, Heartbreak, and Hope*, Warner Books, New York, 1995

Greer, G, 'Obscenity of the Finger Food Feasters', *Guardian*, 6 October 1994

Heller, Z, 'Home Thoughts from the Land of Excess', *Independent on Sunday*, 20 August 1994

Hernandez, A, 'Judy Freespirit', *FaT GiRL* #1, 1994

hooks, b, *Sisters of the Yam: Black Women and Self-Recovery*, Turnaround, London, 1993

Howe, R, 'Style Dictators', *ES Magazine*, 30 September 1994

Ind, J, *Fat is a Spiritual Issue: My Journey*, Mowbray, London, 1993

Jenkins, T and M Farnham, 'As I Am', *Trouble and Strife* 13, Spring 1988

Johnson, A S, 'Anna's Place', *Living Large* 20, September/October 1996

Kelly, 'The Goddess is Fat' in *Shadow on a Tightrope*, (see Schoenfielder, L and B Wieser)

King, M, 'It Can't Be Either' in S Rose; C Stevens, *et al*, *Bisexual Horizons: Politics Histories Lives*, Laurence and Wishart, London, 1995

Klein, R, *Eat Fat*, Picador, London, 1997

Lewis-Smith, V, 'As Advertised by Hugh Grant', *Evening Standard*, 7 July 1995

Louderback, L, *Fat Power: Thin May Be In, But Fat's Where It's At!*, Hawthorne Books, Boston, 1970

Lyons, P and D Burgard, *Great Shape: The First Fitness Guide for Large Women*, Bull Publishing Company, California, 1990

Mason-John, V, 'Keeping Up Appearances: The Body and Eating Habits' in N Godwin, B Hollows, and S Nye, *Assaults on Convention: Essays on Lesbian Transgressors*, Cassell, London, 1996

Meadow, R M and L Weiss, *Women's Conflicts About Eating and Sexuality: The Relationship Between Food and Sex*, The Haworth Press, Boston, 1992

Mennell, S, 'On The Civilising of Appetite', in M Featherstone, M Hepworth and B S Turner, *The Body: Social Process and Cultural Theory*, Sage, London, 1991

Miller, A, 'A Model Speaks', *FaT GiRL* #2, 1995

Nataf, Z I, *Lesbians Talk Transgender*, Scarlet Press, London, 1995

O'Donnell, K, 'Why I Had My Stomach Stapled', *Me*, 10 August 1992

O'Garden, I, *Fat Girl: One Woman's Way Out*, HarperCollins, New York, 1993

Ogden, J, *Fat Chance! The Myth of Dieting Explained*, Routledge, London, 1992

Ogle, T, 'Fat of The Land', *Time Out*, 1164, 9–16 December 1992

Orbach, S, *Fat is a Feminist Issue . . . How to Lose Weight Permanently – Without Dieting*, Arrow Books, London, 1978

— *Fat is a Feminist Issue 2*, Hamlyn, London, 1982

— *Hunger Strike: The Anorectic's Struggle as a Metaphor for Our Age*, Faber and Faber, London, 1986

Otobong, K, 'Fattened by Force', *Trouble and Strife* 23, Spring 1992

Pearson, A, 'Comic Oprah From Weighty Issues', *The Observer Review*, 24 September 1995

Platt, M, 'The Fat Busters', *Guardian*, 16 November 1993

Powter, S, *Stop the Insanity*, Orion, London, 1994

Roberts, N, *Breaking All the Rules: Looking Good and Feeling Great No Matter What Your Size*, Penguin, London, 1985

Royal College of Physicians, *Obesity*, RCP, London 1983

Schoenfielder, L and B Wieser, *Shadow on a Tightrope: Writings by Women on Fat Oppression*, Rotunda, Glasgow/Aunt Lute, Iowa, 1983/1989

Schwartz, H, *Never Satisfied: A Cultural History of Diets, Fantasies, and Fat*, The Free Press, New York, 1986

Smith, H, 'Creating a Politics of Appearance', *Trouble and Strife* 16, Summer 1989

Smith, K 'Space', *Living Large* 15, September/October 1995

Solovay, S, 'the good, the bad . . . and the indigestible' *Fat!So!* #3, 1995

Sontag, S, *Illness as Metaphor*, Penguin, London, 1977

Stimson, K W, *Size Rights: The Disability Debate*, Largesse, Connecticut, 1994

— *The Fat Underground: the original radical fat feminists*, Largesse, Connecticut, 1994

— *Fat Feminist Herstory*, all published Largesse, Connecticut, 1994

Stinson, S, *Fat Girl Dances with Rocks*, Spinster's Ink, Minneapolis, 1994

— *Martha Moody*, The Women's Press, London, 1996

Tolmach Lakoff, R and R Scherr, *Face Value: The Politics of Beauty*, Routledge and Kegan Paul, 1984

Wann, M, 'Fat!So? Manifesto' *Fat!So?* #2, 1994

Wiley, C, *Journeys to Self-Acceptance: Fat Women Speak*, The Crossing Press, California, 1994

Wolf, N, *The Beauty Myth: How Images of Beauty Are Used Against Women*, Chatto, London, 1990

Woodward, H, 'the fatter adventures of supermom #9', *Living Large* 22, January/February 1997

Wooley, S C, 'Psychological and Social Aspects of Obesity' in A E Bender and L B Brooks (eds), *Body Weight Control: The Physiology, Clinical Treatment, and Prevention of Obesity*, Churchill Livingstone, London, 1991

Wooley, O W and S C Wooley, 'Obesity and Women I – A Closer Look at the Facts' and 'Obesity and Women II – A Neglected Feminist Topic', in *Women's Studies International Quarterly* vol. 2, 1979